Praise for *Passing for Thin*:

"A smart, sassy, offbeat, funny-sad account of what [Frances Kuffel] discovered about herself when she went from being a very fat woman to a normal-sized one. Weight-loss programs suggest that happiness comes when fat goes, but Kuffel's clear-eyed account reveals a far more complicated truth."
—*Kirkus Reviews* (starred review)

"An absorbing book, and certainly a brave one."
—*Seattle Times*

"Wrenching, sardonically funny."　　　　　—*Salon.com*

"[Kuffel's] delight becomes yours as you read. Kuffel says that one of the three things that she always wanted to do was to publish a book with her name on it. Lucky for us, with *Passing for Thin*, she's just done that."　　—*The Missoulian*

"An intimate and honest story, as fascinating in its grotesque insight as in its inspirational uplift."　　—*The Onion*

"Brave, funny."　　　　　　　　—*New York Post*

"Kuffel's light, ironic style carries the reader quickly through a difficult, painful, and ultimately delightful story. [Kuffel is] an energized, sassy, and funny writer. Let's hope she keeps writing good stuff like this."　　—*Deseret Morning News*

"Above all, Kuffel tells a great story. She possesses an eye for detail, a knack for dialogue and a remarkable sense of humor in the face of adversity."　　　　—*Publishers Weekly*

"Kuffel is honest enough to see that she isn't everywoman and humble enough to know she doesn't have all the answers."
—*Cleveland Plain Dealer*

"Brutally honest. This will be an easy sell to those wrestling with their own obesity, but most enlightening to the people who love them." —*Arizona Republic*

"Detailed, straightforward and humorous, Kuffel's story is worth reading by anyone who is dealing with problem weight or cares for someone who is." —*Cape Cod Times*

"Kuffel pairs unflinching honesty with a wickedly dark sense of humor in describing her first fumbling introductions to the slender, alien body she is left with after losing half her weight, shining a light on the shared human experience of feeling, at times, uncomfortable in one's own skin."
—*Grand Forks Herald*

"With honesty and a dark sense of humor [Kuffel] describes her becoming comfortable in her own skin."
—*Greensboro News & Record*

"This out-of-the-ordinary book and its smart, dry, sometimes-wicked-but-vulnerable author will have readers in love after the first few pages." —*School Library Journal*

"This book is simply riveting. There is not a woman who's ever carried more than her share of body weight who won't identify with every word that Frances Kuffel has written. Kuffel's journey is rich in wit and wisdom. Her book is a jewel and a must-have for anyone who's ever contemplated improving their body as well as their mind."
—Pam Peeke, M.D., M.P.H.,
Pew Foundation Scholar in Nutrition and Metabolism,
author of *Fight Fat After Forty*, and
NBC *Today* show medical expert

"This is a book that will grab you and hold you in its grip, and break your heart even as it inspires you. Frances Kuffel's memoir is so real, so alive with honesty and clarity, you will never forget it. It is a *Pilgrim's Progress* toward the holy city of thin. Kuffel is our confessional poet of fatness, and the struggle toward fitness, beauty, love. She is entertaining and tough, vivid and funny, in a story of victory that will delight every single reader."

—Robert Morgan,
author of *Brave Enemies* and *Gap Creek*

"Frances has given us a brave and unflinching look into the journey of knowing yourself. Her lessons of self-reflection remind us that we are more than the size and shape of our bodies. Her tenderness and humanity come spiraling through every word and it will leave readers empowered and grateful for their lives . . . as is!"
—Jessica Weiner, actionist and author of *A Very Hungry Girl*
—*How I Filled Up on Life and How You Can, Too!*

"Frances Kuffel set out on a true adventure, navigated the dangers, endured, and emerged transfigured. What makes her tale intriguing is that the terrain in question was her own body and its tyrannies. This is a story for our times from a writer with the language, courage, and experience to tell it."

—Deidre McNamer,
author of *Rima in the Weeds* and *My Russian*

"Frances Kuffel's book is brave and beautiful, full of anguish, gritty determination, and the thrill of emerging from obsession."
—Geneen Roth, author of *When Food Is Love*

"*Passing for Thin* is a heartwarming story of one woman's struggle to overcome a lifetime of obesity. Frances Kuffel is incredibly forthright in sharing the pain and shame of being overweight as well as the courage and determination that she found within her to take charge of her life and control her weight rather than have her weight control her. A 'must read' book for anyone who would be empowered to lose weight by hearing about one woman's personal journey and ultimate success."
—Keith Valone, Ph.D., Pys.D.

FRANCES KUFFEL

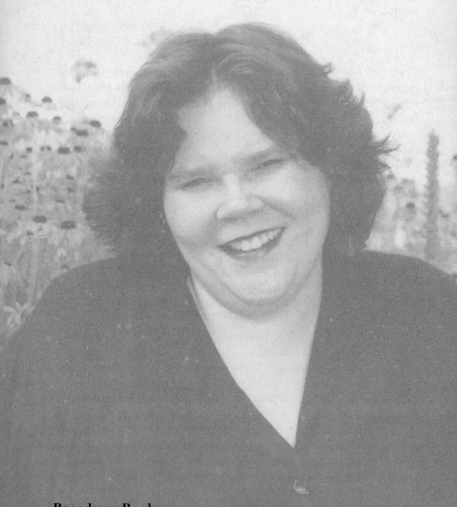

Broadway Books
New York

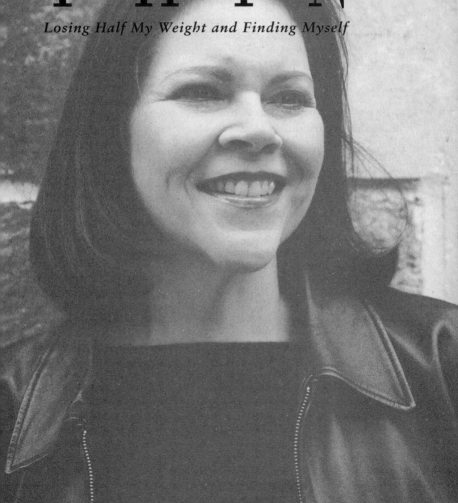

PASSING FOR

THIN

Losing Half My Weight and Finding Myself

To Leonard and Marie Kuffel,
whose hope and charity long outlasted my own,
and to Lisa Kuffel Smith,
whose faith in me began on her first birthday
and who has been teaching me ever since.

There is such a thing as unconditional love.

CONTENTS

1 ARRIVAL ON THE PLANET OF FAT   1

2 LIFE ON THE PLANET OF FAT   21

3 GANGPLANK   39

4 DEPARTURE FROM THE PLANET OF FAT   52

5 ORBITING   68

6 ARRIVAL ON THE PLANET OF GIRLS   82

7 SETTLEMENT HOUSE   100

8 THIS BODY   118

9 HABITAT FOR HUMANITY   136

10 VISIT TO THE PLANET OF FAT   157

11 S.O.S.   172

12 ALIEN VISITORS FROM THE PLANET OF MEN   186

13 CITIZENSHIP   207

14 GIRL OVERBOARD   223

15 AN ALIEN VISITOR TO THE PLANET OF WOMEN   242

Acknowledgments   259

Reading Group Companion   261

"When you wake up in the morning, Pooh," said Piglet at last, "what's the first thing you say to yourself?"

"What's for breakfast?" said Pooh.

"What do *you* say, Piglet?"

"I say, I wonder what's going to happen exciting *today*?" said Piglet.

Pooh nodded thoughtfully.

"It's the same thing," he said.

—A. A. MILNE, *WINNIE-THE-POOH*

PASSING FOR
THIN

1

ARRIVAL ON THE
PLANET OF FAT

No one was there.

I was neither surprised nor unhappy to find myself alone at the Missoula airport. My parents had appointments that morning and had left the arrangements to my brother. Jim was late or the plane was early, it didn't matter. I was glad for the time. I could absorb the difference between New York and Montana. I'd left New York at dawn under its August pall of heat and rusty horizons and emerged into air so finespun it vibrated. The smell of ozone, clover, and cinnamon lingered from thunderstorms the night before, not yet evaporated in the dry desultory heat of midday; the cornflower sky glowed famously big, even in the valley. The Montanans milling around me at the curb were tall and blond, speaking with nasal cadences that, pronounced with a looser jaw, were a perfect west Texas drawl. Conversations there were always, I was reminded again, about the weather. Ask a Montanan about his chemotherapy and he'd give you that evening's forecast. Gaits and gestures were just shy of torpid, the sky and mountains rambled on and on in their own sweet time. Montana was a *slow* place.

I watched the crowd with the furtiveness of a refugee, hoping fervently I wouldn't see anyone I knew. I wasn't ready.

I am five feet eight inches tall, medium framed. That Friday noon I weighed 168 pounds, my lowest weight since sixth grade. I didn't know who or what I was as I braced myself for Jim's arrival. I had one history in that town, a mean one, of being a freak with a brain, allowed to watch but not play. A talking head on a mountain of formless flesh.

In second grade I weighed 115 pounds, by the end of sixth grade, 174 pounds. I lost a proud 36 pounds between my freshman and sophomore years in high school, getting down to 204 pounds. By college I struggled to stay at 248 pounds. I think. Our scale topped out at 245, so I was guesstimating. My top weight of all time: 338 pounds. I had begun this weight loss seventeen months earlier, in 1998, at 313 pounds. More or less—I didn't purchase a scale until the second week of the diet. Jim had last seen me, the year before, 100 pounds heavier.

And so I was glad for this pause, glad for the narrow opportunity of a cigarette, a five-year habit, before being thrust into my assiduously tobacco-free extended family. I was smoking at the curb when I saw Jim hurrying across the parking lot, scanning the clumps of people. Even my big brother's dash across a parking lot roused specters of the things he could do all those years that I could not.

Jim's eyes darted with worry as he paused for traffic. Had he missed me? Had the flight been delayed? He shook his head as he bolted around a pile of luggage, heading in to look for me at the carousel. I tossed my cigarette into the gutter, forming a joke about the life we've shared: *Wanna buzz the root beer stand before we go to lunch?* He walked right past me.

"Jim," I called.

He panned the sidewalk, looked at me, the other people, searching for the voice.

"Uh. Jim? Over here?"

The look—blank.

The second look—questioning. "France? *Francie?* Oh my—wow!" A beat as he took the measure of his reaction, then a conscious modulation. "I'm sorry. I didn't recognize you."

People ask, "Were you always fat?" The photographic evidence is inconclusive.

There is a picture taken for my father's office desk, a studio portrait: my brothers with Brylcreem–slick hair and cotton shirts buttoned up to the necks, my mother looking like Madeline Kahn in black and pearls, me, the baby of the family, front and center in a dotted Swiss confection that must have itched horribly. At two, I fill the dress to capacity, my arms dough-ample and my face full. A year later, a photo shows me sprawled next to Dick, my oldest brother. I'm rangy. My long legs are dimpled a bit at the knees but I'm growing out of the baby fat of that earlier family portrait. A year or so later, I am stalky-legged, my stomach pushes at the buttons of my dress. In this last photo I am intently inventorying the contents of my and my cousin's Easter baskets; she, blond and pixieish, is talking to the photographer.

Once in a while, a photograph distills a truth to its essence. Everything about my next thirty-seven years can be culled from that picture. Fat and thin, my total absorption in food no matter whose it is, and other people's engagement with a world I blotted out.

I identified myself as fat at such an early age that for a long time there was no other adjective to follow. I held the strong suspicion that I was given my serious name because it echoed the word so closely: Fat Frances, Fatty Francie. I hated it. After my mother explained that only boys could be called Junior, I decided I wanted to be named Cathy.

"Fat" is a powerful word to a child. It's one of the first words we learn to read and spell, like "cat" and "dog." It yields similes so easily that it prods the teaser to greater flights of fancy. Where pigs are invoked, whales, elephants, and Sherman tanks are sure to follow.

The average preschooler is not often categorized, with any degree of finality, as mathematical or musical or athletic. She is "cute," "good," "bright." Even disparaging descriptions are carefully phrased for further evolution. "A difficult child." "A plain child." "A clumsy child." "A slow child." I was "fat." A noun, not a modification, to my ears it was my definition and destiny. Not remedial but remediless. It was not a matter of not living up to my potential or being on probation for further measurement, but a fait accompli, an irrevocable pronouncement. Right up there with "crippled," "mentally retarded," or "deformed."

Worse-squared were the terms that came later. One evening, in fourth grade, sitting companionably with my father as he ate dinner after late rounds at the hospital, I picked up a *Journal of the American Medical Association* and flipped idly through it. My father rarely initiated conversation, so questions were a good way to get him talking. "How does penicillin work?" might prompt ten minutes of explanation I didn't understand, but it was hearing his voice that I wanted most.

I paused over a photograph of glistening marbled guck, parted neatly by a retractor to display a cluster of pebbles. "Eee-ewe," I squealed with lascivious horror as I studied the caption. "What does—" I paused to spell out the unfamiliar word "—'o-bee-sess' mean, Daddy?"

" 'Obese,' " he grunted. "That's you."

I knew exactly what he meant. The word tocked across my head like a cuckoo clock. "That's you. That's you. That's you."

The next question I'm asked is why I got fat. It's a remarkably Victorian question, the nexus of Mendel and Freud. Were my parents fat? Is it genetic? The answer "yes" holds the possibility of a kind of forgiveness born of inevitability. *Oh, well, in that case . . .* But my parents were not fat. And I am adopted so I don't know whether this is the trajectory of my forebears or an anomalous burp of biology. Lack of information turns the question to nurture versus nature. I can hear the interrogator's mental calliope churning, *What happened*?

Food happened. Food in conjunction with circumstances. My obesity snowballed. A few motivations for eating—safety, satisfaction—prompted half a lifetime's compulsive eating, which in turn made me a fat girl/woman to the world and a whore to food in my heart. Compare it to alcoholism. If bourbon helped Joe Doe ask a girl to dance one night, does that justify being drunk twenty years later?

Still, people want to know what lay behind the first compulsive bite.

I don't know; I don't remember.

I suspect I had the first bite hardwired into me, that anything could have gotten the snowball rolling. Maybe I wandered into the kitchen after Topo Gigio one Sunday night, and the worm turned. That was the cookie that was one too many, the first of thousands that wasn't enough.

I don't know why I started overeating, but I do know that food was animate, a completely mutual and unfailingly loyal friend. I ate not only because at that particular moment I was bored, but because it had comforted me when I was frightened by *The Twilight Zone* the night before, and excluded from ice skating last Saturday, and bereft when my parents went to a convention in Vancouver last year. My reasons snowballed as much as my weight did. Take any event or crisis and it included all those before it and any I could imagine for my future.

At five-thirty it had been dark for an hour, despite my father's daily announcement that the days were getting longer. Given the afternoon we'd been through they couldn't stay short enough. It was all-hands-on-deck, and we'd been cleaning since we'd gotten home from school. After eighteen months of building and endless finishing touches, our house, in a cul-de-sac of what would be ten classic sixties ranch houses owned by university professors, local business owners, and doctors, was *done*. Green shag wall-to-wall carpets, built-ins straight out of *The Jetsons,* paneling in every room. It was perfect. It was time to have the Monsignor to dinner.

Monsignor Meade was, as far as I could tell, 250 years old. He had been "the Monsignor" when my father went to St. Anthony's in the thirties. No matter was too small for the Monsignor. We all knew the story of how he chastised Dad about his high school girlfriend: "What's the matter, Leonard, Catholic girls aren't fast enough for ye?" He gave thundering sermons (" 'Stacy' is no name for a Catholic baby!"), checked us third graders' collection envelopes, and showed up in school to hand out grades, which he read and commented on. He had baptized me, heard my First Confession, and administered my First Communion the year before. My brothers had gone the same grade school course, as well as serving Mass for him. The Monsignor was known to scold or compliment altar boys on the altar, out loud, forming a crowded congregation's impression of said lad.

So, too, the Monsignor had taken a hand in fashioning my

father's career, informing him that he would join the Knights of Columbus and take his Fourth Degree as a sign that he was a sanctioned Catholic doctor.

No one took this dinner lightly.

"You *will* come in when the Monsignor arrives," my father instructed Dick and Jim. "No horseplay. Afterward, you can go downstairs until supper, but keep it to a soft roar, understood?"

"And put your shoes on," my mother ordered. "Tell them to put their shoes on, Leonard."

"Shoes. On," my father ordered. You could ignore Mom; you risked your ass if you didn't obey Dad. This was not abuse, it was justice. He stated the rules and gave fair warning. We'd each tested him once or twice and never needed to again.

"And double-check your rooms," Mom added, now that she had Daddy's backing. "We'll be giving the Monsignor the tour of the house."

Dick, Jim, and I shuffled off to our rooms for a final inspection. My brothers looked like *Dobie Gillis* teenagers. They were popular and talented athletes with girlfriends and part-time jobs, well-loved jalopies, and letter jackets. The boys and I were bit players in the Dinner for the Monsignor, rounding out the cast of the Happy Catholic Family, but, at seventeen and fifteen, they had their own dramas, downstairs and after dessert. Rosalie and Helen, Scott and Don, shoot-'em-up TV, and Leslie Gore awaited them. I was onstage for the whole shebang, in my green plaid school uniform, properly shod, performing the tasks delegated by my parents, my passions nervily in heat. My affair with food, unlike my brothers' friends and girlfriends, didn't come after anything. It was with me all the time.

I was swooning in the promiscuous smells of company coming. Sterno and the buttery, clean-laundry waft of cheese dip in the chafing dish drifted under the beef Wellington in the oven, layered with carnations and candle wax, Mother's Chanel, and the acrid steam of the dishwasher. Freshly ironed white linen, the cold gleam of Lenox, my grandmother's crystal, the satin swirl of sterling. I loved to put the sugar spoon in my mouth, broad and whorled. It should not be overlooked, in the whys of compulsive eating, that food can be a raw flood of the five senses. My synapses crackled as I waited for the orgy to begin.

"Francie." My father interrupted my flirtations with the Wheat Thins. I was arranging the cold-cut plate by taking care of the broken crackers. "I need you to hold the match."

My shoulder blades pinched. Every night we tested my mettle against Dad's martinis and I flinched as he twisted a lemon peel over the flame. I was pleased to share this ritual with him and by my temerity, and I marveled at how the lemon oil flared, more smells, of burning and citrus, sulfur and juniper. Most of all I marveled at my father. Who else used pyrotechnics so casually?

He turned to mix Mom's Rob Roy next. "Honey," he said, stumped in front of the refrigerator shelves, "are we out of maraschino cherries?"

"We can't be," she said over the grinding beaters. She was whipping cream for the horseradish sauce. "Didn't I get a jar when the neighbors came over last week?"

Frowning with preoccupation, I backed out of the kitchen. It was one of a brace of phrases I dreaded: "I thought we had . . ." "Wasn't there a whole . . ." "I was planning on . . ." I would have a sudden urge to pee or look up the population of Egypt in the encyclopedia. I was gone, vamoose, away from the discussion of if-when-who, taking the box of Wheat Thins and *Little House in the Big Woods* for good measure.

I sat on the toilet and placed one perfect cracker in my mouth, like the Communion wafer, and sucked the salt off, waited for it to soften into goo. My heart settled and my stomach relaxed its clench against accusations. For half a box of crackers, I was occupied against any consequences. I might make it through a second or third repetition of this slow savoring before I stream-munched the rest of the box. I then had three problems: (1) the evidence of the box (toss under my bed for now rather than the bathroom trash), (2) salt-swollen lips and gummy teeth, and (3) the possibility that the Monsignor would turn out to like Wheat Thins as much as I did. Then we'd be back to the awful sentences. *We had a whole box, Leonard . . .*

Thank God for Khrushchev. My mother was prepared for atomic war. From the interstices of the pantry, among jars of stale bay leaves and tins of smoked oysters, another bottle of cherries was found. I helped myself before taking the crackers and mortadella into the living room. My lips were now swollen and a lively cherry red. Years later, I would be tempted to spend money for this look.

My walk-on, as Francie, the Kuffels' Youngest, seen but not much heard, came in the choking duty of answering the doorbell. "Good evening, Monsignor," I singsonged, parroting the classroom greeting. "Please come in and let me take your coat."

He shrugged out of his massive overcoat and handed me his pompommed birretta, before arranging his purple-trimmed cassock with its thousand buttons. "Ahrre ye helpin' yer mother tonight like a good gel?"

"Yes, Monsignor." I staggled off to my parents' bedroom with his coat, the beanie perched on top like a widow hen, holding my breath against crushing it. To do this, I passed the two-foot statue of the Blessed Virgin that my mother had commissioned for the stained glass altar in the entry hall, by the bas-relief of Christ in Gethsemane (a gift from a dying patient) in the bedroom hallway, to my parents' bed, where I laid out the Monsignor's things under the crucifix that cunningly housed holy water and chrism in case of a sudden need of Last Rites. "Extree Munction," I shivered with a delicious gothic frisson. For whom would we need it? The voices were safely three, safely distant. I had time, alone, to dip into Dad's stash of Almond Roca. When saying hello to a guest was a matter of life, death, and afterlife, fuel was called for.

First I scraped the almond bits off with my front teeth,

chipmunk-style. I let the chocolate melt and the toffee soften. Chomp, chomp, chomp—exactly three—and suck the toffee fillings out of my tender new molars. It was a few weeks after Christmas, Dad's stash was full. I took another and this time I was not patient. I went straight to chomp-and-suck.

And so it went. For every task I carried out, there was food to cadge, despite the sad entrée of beef Wellington, the slices calibrated numerous nervous times to feed six diners. I skimmed as I carried out Mom's instructions. A bite of mortadella as I filled the water pitcher; a mint melting on each side of my mouth as I carried in condiments; half a roll squirreled against my cheek, pillow-safe, when I opened the packages for heating, the other half after I shut the oven door. This was Dutch-courage eating. There would be scrutiny passed with the bread basket. It was also the desperate last forage before I had to act like the food didn't matter as much as the company. No seconds of meat would be forthcoming. I couldn't understand why my parents considered this a menu fit for the greatest personage in our lives.

I hovered with each dinner plate, which I'd arranged with its complement of Parmesan roasted potatoes and peas and onions, as Mother carved. I adored those potatoes. Canned new potatoes, they were soft and firm under the skin of butter and cheese they'd been fired in. I left a half dozen in the pan, a wise number. Mom could say, "Yes, we have more but not many," and the request would drop out of deference to the Monsignor's possible desire for another helping. I crossed my fingers and watched as the heels of the roast rocked back (they had too much pastry to serve at the table but that was my favorite part) and my hand shot out to get them out of Mom's way. When she goofed and a slice slid to the floor, the dogs jumped to their feet under the carving board where they were parked, an exuberant tangle of black and yellow Labrador anticipation knocking heads as they untwisted themselves. I was faster, although I nobly allowed them some of the meat. The Monsignor was watching the table attentively as I passed back and forth with the plates. An entire portion of roast beef was a hard thing to conceal in my mouth.

Safely cradled and mollified in the arms of carbohydrates, stimulated just enough from that sleepy place by sugar, maintaining the delicate balance with protein, I was a nine-year-old drunk, as proficient at mixing cocktails as my father. I did not misbehave. I did not fight with my brothers. I did not have any I'm-a-little-teapot moments of showing off. I was helpful, obedient, and absolutely oblivious to the grown-up conversation and dynamics.

The point was to keep getting as much as I wanted without anyone catching me.

My chances increased when I cleared the table. And the plates.

I had no witnesses.

Hence those scraps of roast beef and half-moons of pastry, along with the uneaten potatoes and Parker House rolls that had been "too much, Mahree: ev'rything is delicious, always delicious!" were neatly recycled into me. Even vegetables, the onions a nice counterpoint to the bland bread and potatoes, even *cold* peas. I licked the dessert plates of their whipped cream and graham cracker and walnut crumbs down to the satin china, vanished the evening's beginnings by fetching the chafing dish and cracker tray with its dried and curling cold cuts from the living room where the grown-ups were talking parish business and parish gossip.

The boys careened by to make peanut butter sandwiches, adding to the mess, adding to the food I got to handle. "Too bad, Chunky," Dick snickered. His part was over, he could resume his swaggering. "Stuck with the dishes and kissing up to Monsignor. We get the dogs and we're goin' downstairs."

Jimmie took a jar of jelly out of the refrigerator. "I want to say good night to the Monsignor."

"Well, I know who the *fattest* kiss-ass is, I just didn't know you were the most *pathetic*," Dick said.

Jimmie was one of the Monsignor's favorite altar boys, singled out to teach altar boydom to fifth graders. I sat in on these sessions—he used my old Playskool xylophone to mark the consecrations, and I made fake hosts from Wonder Bread flattened by the heel of a glass. It was one of the few things Jim and I did together besides fend off Dick when he was gunning for both of us at once. Mom always said Jim was the most devout of us kids. Dick was the least but I was there at dinner when he bragged to the Monsignor about playing varsity football for Loyola, and I knew how long it took him to make his confession and say his penance prayers.

"You wanna ask the Monsignor for his blessing, Jim-Wit?" Dick badgered on. "Maybe find out when the Sodality girls are meeting next?" He waggled his blond eyebrows leeringly.

"Ah, Dick, shut up, willya?"

Jim and I froze in place, my hand in the sudsy water, his knife making a faint *ping* as it dropped against the jelly jar.

"What did you say?"

Jim remained silent and still. He was smaller than Dick by a couple of inches and forty pounds, but lots faster. If he got away, we might have a hostage situation on our hands. I wouldn't go down without a fight. My fingers curled around the carving fork in the sink. Pushed to it, Jim and I would, and had, fought Dick with weapons. Broomsticks, forks, sneakers, textbooks, and tennis rackets sometimes slowed him down enough to get away, or cornered him until Dad could sort us out into our demilitarized zones.

I turned my head slowly toward Jim, who said nothing. He was looking blankly at the smeared bread on the counter.

Like a grizzly bear interrupted in a feast of maggots, Dick sensed the motion of my head. Whatever moved had "dessert" written all over it. "What did he say, Chunky?"

"Jimmie wants to say goodbye to the Monsignor," I answered. "Daddy won't like it if you don't go too, and then the Monsignor will want to go downstairs." Jimmie exhaled softly.

I'd saved us. Dick would not want to be responsible for a 250-year-old priest's heart attack. How long would Dad ground him for *that*? I resumed washing up, wondering what I could needle out of Jim for my quick thinking. A ride to Woolworth's? Money for Hostess cupcakes? We'd have a payback skirmish at a time of my choosing, but for now I kept the peanut butter jar in sight.

Did Jim leave the sandwich stuff out for me to clean up after them? Was it his way of saying thanks or mea culpa for the slap upside the head Dick gave me as he stalked off to the living room? I held my temples between my wet hands and pressed hard at the spiraling pain, then let go to drag a finger through the jelly. Mom's plum jelly was winefully rich.

"G'night," Jim said on his way back from the living room, scooping up the stack of sandwiches.

"Don't let the bed bugs bite," Dick smirked. "Although maybe they'd chew off some of your big ass." He tee-hee'd down the hall, a drunken rooster. I took another dollop of jelly, let it dissolve on my tongue as I hefted the carving fork to put it in the knife drawer, wanting to use it, wanting to tell Mom or Dad and knowing I'd get in trouble for interrupting, not knowing what I wanted to tell them, knowing I'd be branded a tattler.

Goodbye, Emily Post; hello, *Lord of the Flies*. Behind the grown-ups' backs we lived in an unpredictable muddle of shifting alliances, imminent violence, and a subtle electric undercurrent of predatory sexuality that our busy parents were not hep to. Dick turned it on Jim and me, leaving us to exorcise the taint (not quite a stain; he didn't go that far) by finding safer harbor in our own ways. My safety was in food.

Or, maybe, it was in being fat. Maybe, very early, I did a very smart thing and made myself as unattractive as possible to Dick's rapaciousness. Maybe that was why I started eating.

Or maybe it was the loneliness I felt when they left for the basement. Dick scared the bejesus out of me and Jim annoyed me, but, God help me, I worshipped them. On rare occasions of truce or necessary alliance, my brothers shared with me their talents for fun—exhilarating, adult-defying fun. The Cat in the Hat would be ham-green with envy for us, although our piles of cousins and more obedient neighbors thought us hellions. We roamed around our summer place on Flathead Lake like banshees, on foot, in boats, and we were untethered from home as soon as we learned to ride our bikes. My brothers showed me that velocity was as polymorphous as food, a million shades of blue and silver, redolent of gasoline and gunpowder, and tasting of sweat and Coppertone. Go fast enough, and the shudder of the boat or Dad's old Citroën worked its way up from my feet to my pelvis to my throat as I joined their howling laughter and crowing glee. They taught me how to curse, how to swim, how to sneak out of the house at night, and how to pee standing up.

I turned to the refrigerator and grabbed Dad's deer salami, bit into it fiercely. I needed to *chew* (not crunch, not dissolve, not masticate like a cow—this was not a carrot stick, Almond Roca, or dinner roll moment) as I struggled with the feud in my chest. I hated them, I loved them, I wanted to be with them downstairs, I wanted to be alone and curled around more food and my book with my chapped teddy bear standing sentry. Food, Teddy, and Laura Ingalls were exclusively loyal to *me*. Food wanted me. I wanted it.

With the hum of voices in the living room, and the carnage of *Gunsmoke* from the basement TV, I retreated to my bed and *Little House in the Big Woods,* making raids as my supplies got low. The challenge was to make it to the kitchen and back to my room without encountering anyone, or of making a convincing case of fetching a glass of water if I did.

A variety of tricks for spiriting food away to eat alone was necessary.

The most obvious was pockets. They had limited space, however, and food emerged covered in lint. All of my pockets sagged and were lined with crumbs.

Underpants were very useful, allowing more and safer cargo space than pockets. My pleated uniform skirt could conceal quite a lot of food. The drawback was itchiness and a short shelf life, as it were. I was eager to divest my treasure quickly, so I didn't want to dawdle or be hung up by conversation.

The stiff-arm approach had two basic positions. If the food was in a box or was loaf-shaped (or, for that matter, a loaf), I held it to my side, either up the inside of my arm or down my leg. I had to sidle by obsequiously, as though I was doing my inspector a favor by getting out of the way. Long loose sleeves were expedient.

Greasy, wet, or sticky stuff was the Olympic challenge of fringe eating. A favorite was the ol' wrap-it-in-a-towel, or item of laundry, so that I seemed to be doing something helpful. If I was particularly adroit, there was a sort of tai chi technique that was a beautiful thing to execute. I held the bowl or plate—wobbly, squishy food, dessert or cereal or noodley stuff (we did not have "pasta" in Missoula, Montana, 1965)—behind my back, nonchalantly swinging it around in the split second I passed a witness. It was too stressful for many repeat performances.

All of these techniques required the closest intimacy with food. I held it tight against my body—on my body—with tender marsupial care.

My favorite fantasy as a preschooler growing up in the Cold War was that an atom bomb would wipe out everyone but me, and I would be left with Missoula's unscathed grocery stores. I knew exactly where I would start: the bakery.

It is such a lovely soft fall, a good starchy jones, a much easier ride than the jagged, energy-scattering sugar high. The best high came in its combo form, not candy but pastries, combining elements of both sugar and starch. Feather-bedded in its easy depth, I calmed and concentrated. Under its barbiturate affect, I could tolerate the teasing of my brothers, the echoing big house. Home was not so lonely when I narrowed the vaults of its emptiness with bread.

Sugar had its attractions, if I needed a spike. I loved, for instance, candy bars at the country club pool, shaking with sun and hunger as the wrapping wilted in my wet hands. Seven-up bars (are these made anymore?) and Planters Peanut Rolls, a satisfying salty descent into the cream center and no chocolate mess, although the peanuts threatened to unglue from the nougat and I would finish with jet streams of salt on my swimming suit from wiping my wet hands. With the candy threatening to dissolve, I wolfed it, fast as fast, before the chocolate became hand cream, too quickly! Oh *why* couldn't I wait for my hands to dry so I could make it last just once?

Food transmuted from pleasure to fantasy, and I had a very active imagination. I ate when I was lonely or bored, not an infrequent condition after my mother found her sweet Lucy in the post-Vatican II kumbaya glory days of the Church. I could make all the promises of the children's canon come true. Food was a flying carpet, Mr. Peabody's Wayback Machine, *A Wrinkle in Time*, the magic wardrobe, *The Secret Garden*.

Books, movies, and musicals were real to me and are forever stamped with the foods they featured. The bare necessities for Prince Christopher Rupert Windamere Vladimir Karl Alexander Reginald Lancelot Herman Gregory James's ball that included six hundred suckling pigs and marshmallows ("for roasting") were just about right. Food *was My Own Little Corner* and Leslie Ann Warren's Cinderella was my kindred spirit in daydreaming. And oh! the heaps of corn and lobster in *Carousel* were a fine thing to visit Maine in search of.

I *pondered* the gustatory exotica of my books. How could I make maple syrup harden as Laura and Mary had in the Big Woods? What were the "sweetmeats" that popped up in "Aladdin and the Wonderful Lamp"? I read "Hansel and Gretel" with the shame of a double agent. I would have eaten the bread rather than mark my path through the woods with it, and I'd have sold my soul to have my way with the gingerbread house.

So, too, I doubted I would offer to carry the Christmas muffins to the Hummels as that brat, Amy, did in her one-upmanship over my heroine, Jo, in *Little Women*. I lusted for and tried to approximate it all: Heidi's toasted cheese and bread (where could I find goat's milk?); the smell of hot buttered toast that "simply talked to Toad" in *The Wind in the Willows*; the chocolate cake bobbing against the ceiling in *Mary Poppins*; Eliza Doolittle's chocolates in a room somewhere; apple strudel, schnitzel, and noodles from *The Sound of Music*.

Julie Andrews may be personally responsible for a good ten pounds of the weight I magically amassed.

It gives new meaning to devouring books.

These emotional contexts were, *all of them*, present in any given bite. When a thing like food is that heavily laden (all the books, all the fun and anticipation of cooking, all the meals, all the jokes and conversation at meals, all the traditions of meals), it takes a lot of it to re-create the import it carries. But the reasons why I ate are much less important than the eating itself, and what it did to my body and my life. The motivations are lost in the food, in my increasing bulk, in my loss of participation. Food wanted me. I wanted it more than I wanted anyone else. That is all that matters.

Another question I am asked: when did I know my eating was out of control?

There was a defining moment. It was idiotically mundane.

I was a thirty-two-year-old assistant in a literary agency, adjunct teaching during the academic year to supplement a salary wildly inadequate to my dependence on restaurant deliveries, constant junk food grazing, and ambitious cooking projects.

For nine months a year, for over ten years, I went from an office to dismal classrooms to teach freshman composition. Weekends were devoted to marking papers and reading manuscripts in the barbiturate haze of starchy carbohydrates. For three months of the year, because I had spent every dollar of that extra income as soon as I'd gotten it, I was frantic.

That summer I was freelancing for an insurance industry newspaper. I eked by, barely.

I had three dollars to my name. A check from the newspaper was forthcoming, that day or the next, and my paycheck was a few days off. There was food in the house, I had subway tokens. I was OK. I knew I was OK. I could lose the three dollars or give them to a homeless person and I would survive. But at eight in the morning I was stricken with panic that I was three dollars away from being homeless myself.

I went out and bought a can of Pringles.

Really, Pringles are a masterpiece in design. They are perfect. Taken in whole, with the curvature of the chip cupping the tongue, they can disintegrate at leisure, consummately savorable. Taken in whole, with the curvature counter to the tongue, they are weapons. I was eating as fast as I could, slicing the fragile gum line along my upper molars, as I called my best friend, Carol, in tears.

"I'm so afraid," I sobbed and spewed wads of spittled chips, which I swiped back into my mouth.

"Do you need a loan? Can you get home? Is it the electricity or something?"

"No," I wailed. "I brought lunch, I have stuff at home. Only . . ."

"Only what?"

"I have a dollar and twenty-one cents to last until that check comes."

"You said you had three dollars."

"I bought Pringles. I'm eating them now."

"At nine in the morning? Did you have breakfast?"

"Yes."

"So why did you buy Pringles?"

"Because I'm afraid. I eat when I'm afraid . . ."

I *heard* this. It was the truest thing I had ever said. This was my heart and my guts talking, every blood cell in my body condensed into five words.

I heard but I didn't listen. I wasn't ready. It would be ten years before I listened and acted.

But I knew.

Jim shook his head.

I didn't recognize you.

I tossed my cigarette onto the pavement with an ironic snort. Lots of times, I didn't recognize myself. We both reached for my suitcase, Jim doing his big-brother guy thing, I wanting to be sturdily unobligated. I won; I knew how the handle pulled out.

"Nice weather," I ventured. Who was it said England has no seasons, only weather? Montana has winter and not-winter.

"It's finally gotten hot," he answered, and hefted the bag into the back of his van, telling me about lunch with the family. He slammed the door shut and looked at me to confirm the plans. That slight movement alerted my primeval little sister antennae. He wasn't gauging how I felt about lunch but how he felt about me.

I took a deep breath. My family was at the restaurant, waiting for me, my moods, my body and face, and my eating. For the first time since I was an infant, they'd be seeing me—Frances, Francie—for what I looked like without the muffle of fat, without the veil of the unhappiness of being fat. There was plenty of unhappiness in me, as well as shaky hope and wobbly confusion, but I could not, for the first time in my forty-two years, say I was unhappy "because I'm *fat*."

I'd been living on a small bizarre planet for forty years, and hope and confusion were part of a new atmosphere. It was breathable but—well, *thin*.

2

LIFE ON THE
PLANET OF FAT

F rahncees," my boss, Barbara, demanded in her sophisticated Parisian accent that hadn't lost an elongated vowel in her
thirty years in America. "I need the *exact* address of the Javits
Center."

It was 1989 and I had been the assistant in her successful literary agency for ten months when Barbara accepted an invitation to speak at a writers' conference.

I looked in the telephone directories, white and yellow. Nothing. I called Information, which, strangely, did not have it either. I asked the other agent in the office, Toinette, who was a
native New Yorker.

She rolled her eyes. "Eleventh Avenue," she said dryly. "In

the thirties. It's not like she can miss it—it's the size of an air-port. Any cab driver will know where it is."

I duly reported this information to Barbara.

She was livid. "I told you, Frahncees, that I need the *exact* address."

I sputtered what I had tried, conscious that my hands were sweating in anxiety. She cut off my explanation.

"You *know* how nervous public speaking makes me. I ask one simple thing and you can't *find* it?"

I swallowed hard, hung my head as I apologized with an-other repetition of what I had tried, what I had been told. She thumped off to Toinette's office.

I had lived for two years in New York City with absolutely no occasion to go to the Javits Center. Had someone told me it was listed under *Jacob* Javits, a name it is never called, the ad-dress would have been forthcoming. I was from Montana. What did I know from dead New York senators?

I got the silent treatment for the rest of the hour she was in the office, which I spent tiptoeing around, cursing my ineptitude, angry at her lack of forbearance. On her way to the door she stopped and stood over me, shaking. "This is not excusable, Frahncees. I had to ask *Toinette* where it is. I asked you to do it."

Not fair! I cried to the gods. Why was she satisfied with Toinette's version and not mine? Despite the fact that I was now crying, I'd had enough. I remembered my mother's advice: al-ways speak in I-statements rather than in you-accusations.

"Barbara," I choked out, "I tried—you heard, you saw. I told you what Toinette told me. I'm sorry you feel I've failed"—my nose was oozing snot, my voice cracking—"but I feel as though"—I was rather proud that I was speaking up for my-self—"I'm being belittled for an effort honestly made."

"Well, you ought to," she answered, or roared, looking down on me in contempt. "You're nothing but a big baby!"

Or did she call me a big *fat* baby? That would be the pot calling the kettle black, since she too was fat. Surely she avoided that word "fat" as religiously as I did.

Thirteen years later, this burns as the most humiliating moment in my life, worse than failing my Middle English exam and losing my teaching assistantship at NYU, worse than a one-night stand telling me it was supposed to hurt, worse than getting my first period in front of the cruelest kid in seventh grade, worse than being deserted on a dance floor in Provincetown when my friend went home for the night with two boys, worse than the note from the man I'd been in love with for fifteen years informing me he was getting married the next week, worse than reading I had become pathetic cameos in novels by erstwhile friends, worse than not being accepted into Cornell's PhD program.

It was the worst because it contained two labels as inarguable and damnable as fingerprints on a pistol. Big. Baby. The omission of "fat" was a mere oversight.

But then all those other moments that point accusingly at my manifold failures since the onset of adolescence can also be laid at the doorstep of being fat.

A functioning addict, I pulled it together for my job. Obesity is weakness made obvious, and I was vulnerable to bias from any direction. Barbara and I chafed at each other. We had many differences of background and temperament I could cite for this, but it really came down to two things: she was accustomed to having servants, and we were both disappointed in ourselves. At thirty-two I was too old not to see the reindeer games, too worldly not to resent them, but I was incapable of leveling the relationship as it lengthened, if not matured. I spent twelve angry years in busy judgment and fear of her.

Why didn't I leave? I tried, once or twice. But, I reasoned, who was going to hire someone who looked like me?

Successful literary agents tend to describe themselves in metallurgical terms. Iron, steel, Teflon. I care most that people *like* me. This attitude is not helpful when I'm trying to please authors, boss, and editors at the same time.

The agent's unglamorous middle ground is in her role as negotiator and bookkeeper; the glamorous parts of the job come in discovering talent (in the unglamorous settings of home, in pajamas or sweatpants), and in lunches and parties and conferences, where she is judged for the dollar-worth of the talent she has discovered. One way to keep the image going is by how she looks.

"Fat Is Beautiful" will never wash. I couldn't believe it then, and I don't now. It may seem unfair, but the fact is that airplane and theater seats are *not* going to get bigger at the cost of profitability, and cholesterol *is* affected by what is eaten and what is burned by the body. The other fact, harder yet and more pervasive, is that people react and dismiss fat people with about as much thought as they give a television infomercial.

A few weeks ago I met a handsome young editor for lunch. He works with a number of men's health and fitness books and I told him some of my story.

"If you'd shown up at that weight," he said, "I wouldn't have respected what you had to say as much."

"Oh, you'd have taken me seriously," I answered rather bitterly. "I would have *made* you. I would have arrived with stories and gossip and obscenities and highfalutin vocabulary and references bursting out of me. I knew I had about thirty seconds to get you past what I looked like." It's more likely I wouldn't have taken him seriously because I would have been so busy performing and furtively snatching bread.

It was a performance I gave twenty times a day. I was good at it.

It was exhausting.

•   •   •

On the Planet of Fat, food was my god, but obesity was my mother, the safe harbor from the consequences of food, offering a reason for why things happened. If I was rejected, it was because of the way I looked or because someone had discovered the fat essence—lazy, dumb, devoid of self-respect and control—of me. And I would never know which of those items was the death knell.

Safe in a body that couldn't do and didn't deserve, year by year I was ceasing to try or earn. Fat infantilized my body, with its pillowy curvelessness and the pudge that made my face ageless. I walked through my days as a child, at the whims of other people's classifications and assumptions and dissatisfactions. With my first compulsive bite, I stopped maturing. I think the reason I have an affinity for children's books, particularly for grade school readers, is that I am essentially eleven years old.

Don't get me wrong. I'd managed a few things not expected of a fat girl from Missoula, Montana, and I wanted things most people want. But obesity is a strict mother. It defines and confines. Everything I have achieved has been in defiance of its definition and confinement of me. At over three hundred pounds, I barely had the physical energy for a job and I was notorious for the sleep I needed.

I had a concise list of what I wanted out of life, three things (my merry mantra): to be thin, to publish a book with my name on it, and to fall in love with a man who loved me back. (In the wisdom of my thirties I revised this to be a *sane* man.) The last two items were predicated on being thin.

I was the prodigal daughter and obesity always slaughtered the fatted lamb when I came trudging home from my failures to live up to my talent or find reciprocity in love. Obesity was Mommy Dearest, forbidding me those things my friends and family took so casually for granted. Christopher was up on Squaw Peak for an all-night cross-country ski under a full moon. Tamara went camping in Hawaii and was invited by brown-skinned, blue-eyed boys to rain forest troves of psilocybin mushrooms. Constance was salmon fishing in Alaska to fund three months in Turkey, mostly naked on various beaches and the Istanbul baths. Kim quit college and moved to New York at nineteen, but thin and pretty, she quickly found a job at Burberry's. It went on and on, my friends' adventures that a reasonable body permitted. Food supplied my adventures. Maybe I would never stand in front of the Angkor Wat myself, but I had Vietnamese delivery on my speed dial.

When my classmates went to Europe or spent the summer reading and experiencing Carlos Casteneda after high school graduation, I asked for a shrink. I read a lot of Shakespeare and wrote precocious poems about suicide. Those were my more productive escapes from the smothering love of obesity.

When I got my master of fine arts in creative writing, my thesis chairman congratulated me. "You're going to make a million bucks, Frances. You're the one."

I promptly entered a writer's block I struggled against for the next fourteen years. I found out why in cleaning a file drawer. In it were a number of yellowed and brittle starts of stories, ideas that came in a flash and seemed destined to write themselves. Holding them, I remembered the thudding urgency, the happy feeling of being a writer, a human role I longed for. When the first spurt was over, I would be hungry, go to the store, and emerge sleepy from the doughnuts or chips or pizza the following day, saying, "Oh well—next weekend." By which time the enthusiasm had withered. I'd lost some essential raw attack instinct that good writing needs to sustain itself. I lost my ability to disappear fully into anything but food, eating to the point of being able to breathe only in shallow sips. In the pincers of that satiation, there is no room for anything except the next tiny breath. I don't do the dishes or throw away the packages. I do not feel whatever propelled me to that state, nor do I have the rationality to consider I may have let myself feed on old feelings in order to have the excuse of eating. I can't even feel regret for what I've done, my whole organism focused on finding a prone position that will allow another tablespoon of oxygen, unable to roll over and having to lift myself in a half push-up as the years-old scarring around my navel weeps and itches from distension. Food is, for me, a fatal disease, and I pine for that locked-down state more days than not.

Dating? I was *fat*. Whether a man I liked would have forgiven me my obesity didn't matter. It mattered to me. The verb "forgive" was the most charitable construct I could imagine for a man's feelings about me. I was careful to disguise my crushes. Raised in a male household, I made friends with men easily. It was my job to keep it looking like I was a pal.

Like a snake in the sun, I am in my most active state around food. I've been high on cocaine and thinking about food. With what could I pleasantly irritate my burning throat (orange juice, nacho chips) and drain my stuffy nose (chili with extra cayenne, Szechwan anything)? What would push this retreat from reality even further?

Obesity's cardinal rule was that anything I wanted I couldn't have, except more food.

Did I really want to be a cheerleader? No. But I wanted the choice.

Small stuff burned as well. One of my oldest friends in New York, Drake, loves to tell me the story of Coney Island, as though I wasn't there. Once upon a hot bright Saturday in the midnineties, Drake and I organized an expedition to Coney Island. Five friends joined us—Dennis, Drake's boyfriend; Toinette, from my office; Drake and Dennis's oldest friend, Sam; Marnie, Sam's girlfriend with whom he was so annoyingly inseparable that I'd nicknamed them Mam and Sarnie; and their friend from Chicago, Lorna. Everyone met at my apartment for Bloody Marys, and Frank and I booked a car-service station wagon to Surf Avenue.

Drake was the King of Coney Island, the Baron of the Board-walk. In all the years and all the fun we'd had—doing off-off-Broadway performance art or voice-overs for his short films, dancing to Tony Bennett at the beach in Rhode Island, getting high on mushrooms on New Year's Eve—I'd never seen him anticipate anything as much as this.

"I love everything about it, Frances. You will too."

"I've seen documentaries," Lorna informed us. We looked at her and waited for more but that was it. For now. She had been informing us on many fascinating subjects for the last hour and a half. European CNN, for instance. The sightings of German U-boats out of Galveston during World War II. How AIDS was decimating American theater. We had begun to stiffen whenever she opened her mouth, and Sam and Marnie were ready to stand *her* up in front of a U-boat.

"You'll all go on the bumper cars with me, won't you?" Drake went on.

"Oh, Drake." Dennis sighed in exasperation from the front seat. My darling boys were not getting along well these days. There was talk of their breaking up. My one bit of family life in New York was slipping away in driblets of bickering and separate passions. Like Coney Island, a concession on Dennis's part, lest anyone forget it.

"I will," I volunteered, and slid down next to him. My butt hurt from sitting on the corrugated floor of the wagon, but I'd volunteered to sit there. The car was packed tight as zipper teeth, and Drake and I were watching Ocean Parkway unspool in the rear window. "I've never been in a bumper car." Drake tilted his grin a little deeper, reducing me, with that grin, to my eleven-year-old alter ego. "As long as I get to ram head-on into

Cookie." He cocked his head and then laughed. Lorna—Lorna Doone—Cookie. We thought that way, in tandem. "But what I really want is to go to the freak shows," I added. "They still have freak shows, don't they?"

"They're all just costumes and makeup, you know," Lorna said.

"Really?" I gasped, wide-eyed. "Was that in the documentary?"

Drake poked my side, his elbow sinking into the folds of my heavy denim jumper and the first roll of fat. "Frances has a crush on the elephant man," he rushed in for the sake of harmony. His mouth dropped in the perfect "O" of Oh-God-I-can't-believe-I-said-that. "And I'm in love with the tattooed lady," he hurried on.

Lorna sniffed in a wind-up for a disquisition on greasepaint and I thumb-tacked over Drake's cover-up, "As long as she's tattooed with the elephant man's name."

Dennis paid the driver as we gathered along the wire mesh fence to get our bearings. Sixty tinny carnival soundtracks descended at once as little kids darted between us. "OK," Dennis said as he gave us our change from the fare. "So we get a hot dog and do the freak shows. Then we'll have a drink, right?"

"Wrong," Drake corrected. "First the Cyclone."

As though he'd said, "First the Sistine Chapel," we all looked up.

It *was* a cyclone. Chittering like goblins eighty-five feet above, roaring as it swooped down and past, teenaged girls screamed to the skim-milk-blue sky. Dennis blanched. Drake rubbed his hands and pulled me and Toinette into the park and ticket line. Sam and Marnie stood aside in a conference of kissing whispers. Their heavy-petting romance was full of these little honey-how-do-you-feel moments.

Sam slid his hand up Marnie's shirt and stuck his tongue, way too obviously, in her ear. Drake and I looked at each other

and rolled our eyes but I could nearly feel it, a hand in the
sweat-damp hollow of my spine, pressing the vertebrae one at a
time, a rough palm warm against warm skin.

"Come *on,* Dennis," Drake called.

"I don't think so," Dennis answered. He shook a cigarette
from his box and squinted at us. "You kids go ahead. Uncle
Den-den will wait this one out."

"Well, *I'm* going," Lorna announced.

"OK!" Drake said.

Marnie and Sam concluded their mash-conference and
joined the queue, arms wrapped around each other. "This is
gonna be scay-ree, isn't it?" Marnie said nervously, eagerly, using the drama to drip Mississippi from her voice. She sounded
like she'd guzzled a jar of tupelo honey.

Girls in stone-washed denim jeans and pastel T-shirts
clutched each other or their boyfriends as they wobbled away
from the cars, bragging and tall-taling the terrors above. The
line began to move and we sorted ourselves out to take our
seats. Sarnie and Mam together, of course, then Drake and I
handed our tickets over.

"Nope," the attendant pronounced, looking me over. "It'll
never fit."

"*What?*" Drake asked, askance.

It?

"The safety bar. We'll never get her in."

Her?

"It's OK." I took a deep breath and stepped away from the
gate. "You go."

"You've got to be kidding," Drake protested to the carnie.
"Look, she can sit alone. I'll—"

"Nope. No can do. Rules is rules on this ride."

"Well, that just sucks," Drake said.

"It's *OK*," I spat. "I'm going to go smoke with Dennis. We'll
wave."

"Sit with me," Toinette said to Drake. My mouth pursed.

Five feet two, skinny and tidy in her knee-length Gap shorts, Toinette was my senior at work. Five days a week I felt like a retarded Jolly Green Giant around her.

"Sure," he said, looking at me apologetically. "Of course. It's just that—"

"Let's get loaded up," the attendant said, holding out a grimy hand for the tickets.

"I'll stay with Frances," Lorna said. I blinked back the urge to smack her. I needed to let my cheeks cool, find the joke I could use about being banished from the Cyclone. I needed Dennis's sarcasm for the outing we'd signed on for. After a nasty glare at her, I turned on my heel and crossed the sawdust midway to Dennis, excreting the determined smile of a prom reject taking a seat on the gymnasium bleachers.

"I'll buy ya a beer," I said without pausing, and shied off to the nearest stand.

I came back with three longnecks to a stilted silence. Lorna must have been filling Dennis in on the sensible rules of how the world works.

Dennis took a sip, peered up at the loop-de-loop that Drake, Toinette, Marnie, and Sam were screaming through. "It makes me sick looking at it."

"It makes my back hurt," Lorna added.

I took a long pull of Bud. "I used to love carnival rides."

"I gained some weight once," Lorna said. It was only half a pronouncement.

"Really."

"Not that much, of course. Not so I couldn't ride the roller coaster."

"Ah."

"But it was awful."

"Yes."

"Maybe you'll lose it one day. The weight. Maybe you'll come back and ride the Cyclone."

"Maybe." The burning in my throat was spreading across my

chest, alcohol or embarrassment. The wooden tracks jounced mightily as the train rumbled to a halt. "I think I'd love that roller coaster."

"Oh sweet Jesus," Dennis snapped. "Who'd fucking want to? Look at this place. It's Cairo with clown faces, for fuck's sake."

Maybe. Maybe it was the tawdriest place in the five boroughs. But I liked it—liked the girls in their awful pink T-shirts with their names spelled out in glitter, liked the boys in tight pants, the fat children bawling for cotton candy, the hard-bitten carnies and the smell of popcorn and urine and machine oil in the afternoon heat. It felt authentic. Everybody knew who they were, what they wanted to do next.

"Oh, Gawd," Marnie crowed as they came tripping up. "Was that fun, or what?"

So much fun, apparently, that Drake and Toinette had circled back in line. Dennis sighed impatiently at the delay.

"Once is enough for us," Marnie went on. "Hoo-wee. It was fun, though."

Sam scuffed his yellow sneaker in the dust, looked sheepishly at Marnie. "I want to ride again, too."

"I'll come with you," Lorna said with a quick glance at me. "I don't want to miss out."

She and Sam dashed off to join Drake and Toinette. Time for curly fries.

"Guess we're just sticks in the mud, Frances," Dennis said, taking a fry.

"More like a redwood," I said harshly. "Stick me in the mud and there's no mud left."

At least I had lunch to look forward to, and a hundred vendors to choose from. Two chili dogs and cheese fries at Nathan's with everybody else, followed by a chocolate ice cream cone while the gang rode the Whirl-I-Gig, corn on the cob as we debated having our fortunes told. I slowed down before we headed to the freak show to see the two-headed baby in a jar, nervous about eating in front of the Fat Lady, but I wandered off for roasted peanuts when Drake started competing for a lime-green poodle he'd set his heart on. He and Toinette argued good-naturedly over the correct dart-throwing stance until finally she slapped down a dollar and took a shot as well. Neither won but a new alliance had been forged up in the sky, on the Cyclone. *What else is there?* Cotton candy was too insubstantial, candied apples too gooey in the heat. Tacos? Frozen bananas? I volunteered to get another round of beers and bought a big bag of popcorn to share. "I'm stuffed," Marnie drawled in three or four syllables. Lorna shook her head. "It seems like we've been eating all day."

We stood at the corner of the gaming kiosk as the afternoon deflated around us. The merry-go-round was pinging the same chattery nursery songs it had when we'd climbed out of the station wagon, the smell of clams was nearly visible in the humidity.

"Let's go up to the boardwalk," Drake said. Relief rippled through us. Someone was in charge.

It was cooler there. Clouds were rolling in from the south, bringing a breeze and making the cruise ships' stately progress toward open sea crisp on the horizon. We sank gratefully to the benches.

"There have been a number of fires here," Lorna started in. Sam and Marnie jumped up in irritation and zoomed off to listen to the fifties band blaring down the way. "There was," she recounted, ticking off her fingers, "Dreamland, of course, and—"

"Luna Park, Steeplechase, and *then* Dreamland," Toinette snapped. "We know." She looked at Dennis meaningfully. They shared a habit of having "information." Drake and I could get prickly when they started in but today it was Lorna's turn to annoy. At least Toinette had snippets of stories to go with her encyclopedic memory. Dennis closed his eyes against the tension and stretched out his long legs, lifting his face to the marbled light. The water had a narcotic effect on Dennis. He was always sweeter for it.

"Can you believe what those ladies are wearing?" Drake laughed, getting up to take a look at the obese sunbathers in bikinis. "You can't even see the fabric with all that fat hanging down."

"They look happy enough," Dennis said.

"Ha," I choked. If they were happy, they shouldn't be. They had no right—*none*—when I was stifling in thick denim, my underwear wet through with sweat. I hated them, and, for a bad spasm, I hated anyone who didn't share my hate.

"Maybe they're polar bears," Toinette added. "The Russians out here swim in January." She held up her Budweiser, a signal the afternoon really was falling apart. We were tired, and tired of each other. Sam, Marnie, and Lorna were meeting friends at a jazz club that evening and Dennis was yawning for a nap that would revive him enough for his favorite piano bar. Toinette had a birthday party to go to. Thoughts of a lingering Saturday night preyed on me. Did I have the energy to cook, or should I order out? What did I want? Hot dogs? Nathan's had been good, the fragrance as vast as the Ferris wheel towering above the stand, and it had been fun sitting there together, laughing about the years we'd known each other, the things we'd done, the beach houses we'd shared. Yes. Oscar Mayer franks. I'd make coleslaw, with mayonnaise and sour cream, Ben & Jerry's Black Forest after. An expansion of the day I'd hated and loved.

"You want to hang out some more?" Drake asked me.

"Maybe get another beer?"

"We could play pool." He nodded toward a barn of a place, open to the darkening sky, empty pool tables and empty stools. Our kind of hangout.

"I'm a terrible pool player," I warned him.

"So am I."

Another gust of wind burst off the sound, lifting my jumper skirt. My plaid shorts flashed brightly in the douring light.

"What are you wearing, Frances?" Toinette asked, flicking my hem up.

I shushed her hand away from my body. "Shorts."

"Under your dress?" Drake asked. "Why not just wear shorts?"

"No one will ever see me in shorts. Ever."

"Why wear them, then?"

I looked out on the silver-tipped water. "Umm—modesty? In case the Cyclone blew my skirt up." *That should do it,* I thought. The Cyclone would shut them all up for years to come, a weapon of guilt and sympathy.

It wasn't modesty. Wearing my denim jumper, the coolest item I owned, on a hot day would have chafed my thighs raw for a week to come had I not protected them. Diaper rash at the age of thirty-seven. My shame came layered in shame.

An hour later, I was rambling on to Drake. "I really wanted to ride the Cyclone."

"It's horrible they didn't let you." He bobbed his head over the bar. He was soused.

"And then you rode with Toinette. Do you like Toinette better than me?"

"No, but don't ever tell her. She's so—"

"Know-it-all?" I finished.

" 'Course after Cookie . . ." His eyebrows shot up.

" 'Cause I love you, you know. I feel like we're brother and sister. I could tell you anything."

"I know," Drake said, and put his arm on my shoulders. "I can tell you anything, too. I love you."

"I was really looking forward to the Cyclone."

Missed carnival rides separated me from my friends, and I worried that I shamed them. In that big body I watched and commented, taking up enormous social space in one-on-one interactions. I reported and fractionated my unhappiness and depression, sometimes linking it to my size but not to eating. I lost friends: either they became too busy or I became too much for them. My depression was static and boring. I wearied people.

What I didn't consider was that those friends who remained loved me, and that they were worried.

Drake ends the Coney Island saga by recounting another day we spent together. "When I really got scared for you was the time we went shopping and you were wheezing—*wheezing*—to keep up. I was like, is she gonna do a John Candy on me?"

That's the big stuff: John Candy, Mama Cass. It threatened my life.

At 338 pounds, I couldn't stand for more than ten minutes before my left thigh went numb. Housework or a few hours of Christmas shopping meant I might not get out of bed the next day. At thirty-one, I had abdominal surgery to remove my gall bladder and a thirty-six-pound ovarian cyst. I didn't know I was swollen, as my surgeon told me later, to the size of a nineteen-month pregnancy. I didn't see it. It took a stranger in an elevator to pat my belly and ask me when I was due to prompt me to go into a bathroom and lift my dress, only to discover the misshapen mass. Gallstones and gynecological problems (heavy bleeding, long periods, and painful cramps) are among the classic effects of obesity, along with high blood pressure (which I was prone to), diabetes (my blood sugar flirted with it), cardiac problems (ibid.), and a host of other illnesses.

Fat people take nothing in the material world for granted. Summers begin in April, rivulets of sweat forming humiliating trails of damp on unupholstered seats. Ask a fat man how he feels when he sees a molded plastic lawn chair. It can melt under too much weight, the legs squooshing into the grass or bandying like a cowboy's. When an obese woman is ushered into a guest room featuring an antique bedstead, or gallantly offered a man's jacket on a chilly night, she will insinuate herself onto the mattress, proffer assurances that she isn't cold. A fat person doesn't *fit* the human comforts and imperatives of rest and warmth. What's left? The other necessity of biology—food.

There are hundreds of such moments of being obese among the thin that burn, a verb that describes the landscape of the Planet of Fat. There are other verbs from the Language of Fat:

Endure: The blood pressure cuff that didn't fit, the several attempts with a butterfly needle in my hand because the veins in my arms were inaccessible. Doctors' and hairdressers' gowns that didn't close. Not being able to sit back in a restaurant favored by HarperCollins editors because the Monkey Bar's curved pea-green velvet chairs did not accommodate my breadth. The tops of pantyhose around my thighs rather than at my waist.

Plan: Make those airline reservations early in order to secure an aisle seat where I could spill. (Always, I thought of my excess flesh as spilling, as though I were a toddler deep in SpaghettiOs, as though I were a colostomy bag overflowing.) Have enough money for cab fare because my back will be aching from standing in line at the movies. Take off the skirt and T-shirt to go quickly into the frigid water of Flathead—*now, quick*—when heads are turned or the beach is deserted.

Compress: *Never* swing my arms when I walk. *Always* hang back in doorways to let other people go ahead. Tuck my head to my chest and curl my shoulders and wrap my arms across my chest to minimize the protrusion of my breasts—especially in theaters, and on airplanes, where I would read with one arm clutching the other, book tensed in front of my face for the seven-hour flight from New York to Montana (talk about endurance). Squeeze into the back of group photographs so only my head would show.

Ignore: The glares when I couldn't help taking up too much room. And, hey, the stain on my tits from that lunch at the Monkey Bar?—it could happen to anyone. This editor won't know how often it happens to happen to me. The fact that I had seen Montana through binoculars but had never gotten much beyond the scenic viewpoints, never been intimate with them. Ditto much of New York City, which requires walking and money I needed for food, taxis, air conditioning.

Rage: As quietly as possible at the love I'd missed, the children I didn't have, the countries I hadn't explored, the pointe shoes I never danced in, the jobs I couldn't take because I couldn't stand on my feet that long, my friends as they tossed up everything to move to Tokyo or have a lesbian fling or take up weight lifting or write a screenplay or strip the wallpaper down to the original wood.

Hope: That the subway would have two seats at the end of a row so I could spill both ways. That the train would have benches rather than bucket seats. That the nurse wouldn't mutter my weight under her breath, that the hairdresser would have capes rather than robes. That I could murmur my request for a seat belt extender to a seasoned stewardess. That she wouldn't yell up to the other stewardess after the demonstration.

Hope, even, that someday I would stay on Monday morning's diet for a long, long time. Long enough to get thin.

3

GANGPLANK

Every once in a while I was reminded that I had a body. Located somewhere beneath my brain pan, it was a funny useful thing I could surf straight to glory.

And glory permitted that rarest of commodities—wide-awake hope.

Fourth of July weekend, 1996. I was visiting my brother Dick's oldest daughter, Lisa, and her husband, Tim, in Minnesota. Born five days after my birthday, Lisa was my thirteenth birthday present, as much my sister as my niece, as much my mother as my daughter. We take care of each other and discuss as matters of fact our weird fetishes. It doesn't shock me that she eats bouillon cubes, funfetti after a jelly bean high. She finds the way I talk out loud to myself and my notebooks of lists of things to do the demented but harmless hum of a bumblebee. We laugh that when I am decrepit and still single, she will be the one to change my diapers. Of course, I have to give extremely good birthday presents in the interim.

We had spent two days wandering the shops of Duluth and driving up the shore of Gitche Gumee, dissecting the two sides of our families. On the third morning I mentioned I'd always wanted to go rafting. Tim's ears pricked up. Rafting, now *there's* a project! Lisa and I cast amused looks at each other as he began flipping through the Yellow Pages. He was notoriously telephone-phobic, and except when he was running or skiing, he was the most passive man I'd ever met. I was about to be hoisted on my own petard, and Lisa with me.

How bad can it be? I thought as we set out an hour later. *Rafts like waterbeds, Longfellow's pleasant water courses, maybe piña coladas.*

Lisa informed me that the St. Louis River is where the Olympic kayaking team trains. I watched the root-beer-colored river roll past with distaste; I was used to the clean waters of Flathead. This looked foul, worse than the East River around Brooklyn's decaying dockyards. But there was nothing scary in it. I was looking forward to a pleasant, pretty afternoon.

I argued against the life jacket. "I'm an excellent swimmer," I assured the wiry guide. "Nothing can sink me."

I tried cutting a deal. "I won't fit in your life jacket, so let me sling it over one shoulder, or sit on it."

"Insurance," he said, shaking his head. "Don't worry, we'll get it on."

By the time we packed me in, I felt like a paraplegic. I could barely turn my head and my arms couldn't lift past my shoulders. People stared as we struggled to fasten it; I could feel their prayers that I wouldn't be in their raft.

Instructions were issued by boys in kayaks once we were on the water. I quirked an eyebrow at Lisa and Tim. We're doing this ourselves? Our paddles aren't accessories? No rum drinks? Also in our raft were two giggling young women from the Twin Cities. Lisa was behind me, a former competitive butterfly swimmer, and Tim had taught canoeing. We had their upper-body strength on our side. I sat in front and the last words given before we paddled into the current, "When someone falls out, just haul 'em in: we'll sort you out later," steeled my determination. I could not be hauled aboard. At best, I'd hang on to the end of some raft, slowing it down until I was bashed by the rusty water against a rock. I would do anything to avoid this.

From the dock, the broad river was picturesque with foam but as the current swept us beyond the rafting company's bay, I learned how naïve I had been. We had entered a corridor right out of Stephen Hawking, the event horizon sucking all matter into its maw. The rafters' instructions were dress to get wet, not dress to die.

"Lean *in* to the rapids," the guides shouted back to us as we approached the first cauldron. The mud-colored river was no longer laconic with silt. Iron ore turned it brown, and cliffs roiled it into an iron-fisted thing that tossed us around like a Frisbee. Lisa was muttering, "I don't like this. I don't like this at all," as Tim gave calm directions. Our side of the raft guided our course. The girls simply couldn't balance Lisa's muscles and my terrorized 330-pound resolve. Tim had to paddle on both sides to keep us from going in circles.

Bump! We were in a pile of white water choking out a million different currents, the river wall threatening from behind two feet of chaos. I leaned—*in*—for dear life, and it worked. It was as if someone threw our carnival ride into neutral, giving us the chance to nose out toward midriver and something like tranquility.

"This is your fault we're here, Franny," Lisa wailed.

"It's OK," Tim said, as peaceably as if we were tangled up in a new knitting stitch. "Just do what they say. Francie, keep leaning."

Later I puzzled out the physics involved. By pressing into the water and cliff faces, my weight slid the raft backward, allowing Tim and Lisa enough purchase to nudge us around the worst of it.

I was an amazing leaner. I'd been a leaner as a kid, sailing Flathead. With the black water of a storm approaching, we'd stay out anyway, the daredevil Kuffels, addicted to speed and risk. I was the wild card of ballast. Flathead is a big lake, the winds funnel out of the mountains crazily and storms pack a punch. Flathead, too, has its share of rock outcrops and sucking currents and crushing waves, I was reminded. I'd survived such mayhem before. "C'mon, Lisa," I yelled over the tight cuff of the life jacket. "We're rodeo gals, remember? Yee-haw!"

And so I paddled, deep and hard, and I leaned, the margin of control we needed to keep all parties aboard. Lisa was the powerhouse, Tim was the captain and finesser, the girls—I don't know what they did. By our third rapid we despised them through an unspoken wolf pack vibe. Once, Lisa and I rowed backward to keep us in place so Tim could pull someone aboard. The rescuee lay on the floor of the raft, panting "Oh-my-god-oh-my-god," and Lisa and I redoubled our determination to, if not remain dry—that wasn't happening—remain in the goddammed boat.

And we did. We were the only raft that didn't lose a passenger. The long trip to the beach, across the St. Louis's finally calm waters, was wearying. *Now* could we have those rum drinks?

Ashore, Tim, Lisa, and I were a blast of cockiness and exhilaration. *We* didn't bail anyone, we told the other parties as we soggily boarded the bus. Nope, not us. Their faces told us they found this hard to believe. I looked such an unlikely candidate for survival. But we were bull riders, Neptune's favorites. We kicked ass.

And I—the Pillsbury Dough Girl—had kicked ass. I'd forgotten I had that determination in me. It had been twenty-five years since I'd been a party to daredevilry. I liked it. I wanted more.

To get it in other flying matters—snow, my feet, sex, mountaintops—I'd have to lose weight. A lot of it. It was a reason.

I had never been so high in my life.

1997: I spent the three days after Thanksgiving in bed, exhausted and eating leftovers from the dinner party I had given. Dennis had told me about a movie he'd seen that summer. "It's *sweet*, Frances," he said with rare winsomeness, "a Real F.G." "Feel good"—our shorthand for walking away with goofy saccharine smiles. Three months later it was on pay-per-view. For all its froth, *The Truth About Cats and Dogs* was another siren call to the Planet of Girls, this one speaking to something tender and wistful in me. I watched it twice, heaved myself out of bed to buy a blank tape and record it, watching it again and again.

Questions formed as I ate all of the second of the pecan-sweet potato pies.

I don't always side with underdogs and sidekicks. Jane Austen's Emma Woodhouse annoys me, I took Alex's part in *Fatal Attraction*, I can watch Julia Roberts grin through anything. On the other hand, Melanie is infinitely more interesting than Scarlett in *Gone With the Wind* and I always root for plucky Elizabeth Imbrie over silver-spoon Tracy Lord in *The Philadelphia Story*. There's no rhyme or reason for these preferences. They belong in the category of "just because."

But *The Truth About Cats and Dogs* was different from my other tastes in the chick œuvre. Everyone in the movie admits that Abby Barnes (the invented über woman Janeane Garofalo and Uma Thurman take turns inhabiting) is a superior woman. "Funny, smart, nice," Brian-from-Venice describes her radio persona. Uma Thurman's Noelle admits a little jealously that he and Abby are obviously a match, observing how well they talk together. Even Abby, panicked with insecurity, has an objective sense of her star qualities, which are absolutely aligned with Brian's. Smart, funny.

Hmm, I thought as I ate cold stuffing. *Smart, funny, professional—these were the things that got Brian-from-Venice's attention. Interesting. He liked what Abby knew and how she sounded.*

There is such an emphasis on talk in the movie. "Articulate" is the second adjective applied to my heroine. The radio, the phone, reading aloud, walks-and-talks. I was struck how single words stood out in the dialogue, pronounced as though the characters understood exactly when a word was ripe for the picking.

I lay sappily in bed for three days mulling over Brian's justification that he fell for Abby not for her beauty but for who she was. Maybe fairy tales could come true, even for "ugly" girls.

Even for girls like Abby, who confessed her "freshman forty" to Brian-from-Venice in their not-long acquaintance.

That confession was more than an anecdote. It was Alienese for shame that had not been outlived, a self-perception of "fat" that still haloed Abby in her mirror, and the capacity for gaining it all back.

Janeane Garofalo would be dwarfed in a lineup with Julia Roberts and Andie MacDowell, and she doesn't have the cuddly "Girl I Marry" femininity of a Meg Ryan or a Cameron Diaz. Renée Zellweger complained that it took her many months to lose the seventeen pounds she gained to play Bridget Jones while Hollywood buzz makes a big deal out of Janeane Garafolo's size, which is several labels smaller than the national average. Garafolo is a woman who knows what it is to be slightly slighted for her body. But she *is* gorgeous, especially under careful scrutiny. Brian-from-Venice sees it when he lifts her photograph from the developing solution, sees her contemplative, risk-taking eyes. "Beautiful" includes Janeane Garofalo's eyes.

If.

If. If my body was normal, mightn't other things about me . . . ?

Janeane Garofalo gave me something tangible in my curiosity about the Planet of Girls. You could be smart, ironic, crabby, and a Real Girl. You don't have to be a pipe cleaner to be thin and beautiful. You could inspire the insipid and defy the smug. It wasn't the sunset kiss that got me; it was the long passionate phone conversation before. Abby Barnes and Janeane Garofalo got me thinking. I needed a role model. They gave me hope.

Dennis was, it seemed, getting it together. After the breakup with Drake, he'd pulled himself out of a lingering depression, refurbished his apartment, and was doing things to meet men—going to readings and lectures, date nights at a gay bookstore, to the bars where older men congregate. He mentioned, as we made Thanksgiving dinner for friends and listened to Broadway musicals at full blast, that he had a date the next week.

I ruminated on this for an hour or two before casually saying, "I hope when you get a boyfriend you won't forget me. I'll be out there in Brooklyn with nothing to do and no life." I was half joking. I'd been dumped before when friends fell in love or went on to new interests—it had been months since I'd seen Drake, who had a new boyfriend and was laying low in his fragile first year in recovery from alcohol addiction. I did not want Dennis to be one of those who forget their sad-sack friends when they fall in love.

"Oh, Frances," he said in that way of his—exasperation and empathy, one of his most dangerous combinations. He understood me too well and knew that need can overwhelm when it demands that *a* friendship become *the* friendship.

With company due to arrive soon, he let it slide until January, when he invited me for drinks and dinner at a downtown lounge, Fez. We scored a settee under a camel saddle, Dennis ordered us Stolichnayas, and turned to me.

"I need to talk to you about what you said at Thanksgiving."

I drew a blank until he reminded me of my comment. It came back to me with a soundtrack. "The Simple Joys of Maidenhood" had been on in the background.

"How," he went on, biting the words off like dangling threads, "Could. You. *Think*. I would stop being friends with you? Do you *realize* what that says about *me*? Do you *think* I have no *loyalty*?"

I had to admit his umbrage was justified.

"Further. *If—when*—I meet someone, you've put me in a position of feeling guilty because of *you*. That's not fair."

I nodded and swallowed hard. "I'm sorry," I said, and I meant it.

"What does it say about *you*? Do you think so little of yourself that I would just *drop* you? Do you think we've been friends all these years because I didn't have anything *better* to do?"

I blinked back tears of gratitude. I may have forced the issue, but here was Dennis raising a flag on the North Pole of our friendship.

More Stoli was served and he began to slur as he launched into that night's alcoholic performance, battering me with vodka-greased insights into what it meant to be me—to be adopted, to be obese, to be a literary agent, to live in New York and pine for Montana. It was unending. My tears turned from unearned gratitude to fury to humiliation to disagreement to more fury.

I rarely fight. When verbal fisticuffs are raised I get quiet, especially when I'm blindsided. My brain cramps, my body begins to leak. Not just tears, either. In first grade, when Sister Mary Marcilia had scolding to dole out, she would send me to the bathroom. Dutifully and dryly, I would sit on the toilet, then return to class and the chiding someone was getting, and promptly pee in my seat. When I was sent to the lavatory, everyone else braced for trouble. So I sat and listened and squirmed and leaked. He went on. I was as deep in the vodka as he but I wasn't drunk. I almost never got drunk. It was hard, at 338 pounds, to get liquored up. My recourse to Dennis's litany was to retreat periodically to the restroom to bawl, returning to the ongoing lecture. I ordered Fez's highly unsatisfying pizza, hoping food would help one of us. It didn't. I hailed a cab and took my stumbling Judas home, then backtracked to Brooklyn.

I disconnected my telephone the next day, cowering in bed. I didn't want to hear from Dennis. I was humiliated for us both.

Drake called me at the office on Monday. "What happened? Dennis is in a panic. He called last night and said he couldn't get hold of you. 'I'm afraid I lost Frances as a friend.' Those were his exact words, but he can't remember the details."

"Good," I answered shortly. "I want him to have his dignity."

Dennis was my best friend. At his best he was dazzling in his ability to make connections. I'd heard him mesh Frank Lloyd Wright and *Ferdinand the Bull* in lucid illustration of the architecture of Almodóvar's movies, and he could do so partly because his heart had been broken somewhere. He feinted aside a sad and secret trove of the not-enoughs: not handsome enough, not ambitious enough, not talented enough, not kind enough. Addicts' lists of failures are endless, leaving one or two attributes that are sometimes up to scratch and which are mortally honed with overuse. Dennis could also be warmly rescued by a great *frico del fattore,* a Nancy Mitford biography, or a ribbed cotton sweater. I'd been privy to many moments of surprised pleasure with him, but the night in Fez exposed us both. I now knew what he thought of me, unedited by sobriety. Drake's twelve-step perspective had no hesitancy in pointing out his ex-lover's alcoholism, to Dennis's prickly exasperation. Dennis's suspicion of what he'd done must have been prodigious to call Drake.

"He got gutter-drunk and he set out to shame me. We're still friends. But I'm tired of his drinking. He's got to stop." Drake sighed in response. We'd both been victims of Dennis and vodka's mean sides, and we'd both been spellbound by his charm and urbanity. The two sides were an ice cube apart.

Drake and I had a joke in the bad old days when we were a heavy-drinking threesome. After the second vodka, Dennis would morph. It might take the form of dwelling on a single pointless idea: "Is the waiter gay? He's cute, and too young, but do you think he's gay?" or "I don't care how 'accent' is pronounced. It's just not *right* to say 'flack-sid.' " During these insistent returns to what was not interesting to begin with, we waited for him to implode, his posture wilting as his eyes rolled and he fell silent. Or he could turn vicious, taking us down in turns. It didn't matter which drunk Dennis turned into. We could see the "click" and Drake and I would look at each other and quote from *The Boys in the Band,* "turning." By his fourth drink, we had to get him into a cab with specific instructions to the driver. When Dennis didn't have shepherds at that fourth drink, anything could happen. One Sunday I met him at the movies and was shocked to see his face a mass of bruises and scabs. He shrugged. He'd gotten drunk, didn't know how it happened, had lost his wallet. "Lost it or had it stolen?" I asked. He shrugged again. It didn't seem to matter whether he'd been beaten up and robbed or gotten careless and fallen down. For Dennis, such scenarios were also an ice cube apart.

Dennis and I made up, of course. He came out to Brooklyn that weekend, arriving with two near beers and the announcement that he was changing his drinking. He'd read a book—Dennis had spent fifty years looking for his version of Huey, Dewey, and Louie Duck's one-book-answers-all bible, the *Junior Woodchuck Guidebook*—that called for a month's abstinence from alcohol and then a certain amount each week, calculated on weight, height, frequency, and timing.

"That's great!" I said. "It's like me joining Weight Watchers. I mean, I don't have to give up sugar—I just have to control it." We had our near beers and went off to dinner, happy with ourselves, each other, and the certainty that the Emerald City was a hop, skip, and song down our Yellow Brick Roads.

A week later another friend called with a tale of dinner at Dennis's house. It ended badly, she reported, in a drunken monologue about me. "She has to lose weight," Dennis kept repeating. "She has to stop eating."

"And I suppose he's sharing these insights as he's picking up the empty wine bottle every few minutes to check if there's more," I snapped. "Was he watching your glass? Did he drink the last of it? *I'm* the one with the problem?"

Outrage became my companion that week. How *dare* he? How the *fuck* dare he?

I spent President's Day weekend very close to home. I wasn't particularly "bingeing." This is a term I don't generally use because I ate so much so steadily that it would be hard to isolate the peaks. But certainly I was eating, a lot. I needed to deposit my paycheck, a ten-block round-trip walk. I dreaded how my feet, hips, and back would ache so I procrastinated all the way to Monday evening. I was also thinking about Weight Watchers, down on Montague Street, wondering what their hours were.

I'd been on thousands of diets, self-imposed or the sign-up kind, a new one every Monday. There were—oh, I don't remember them all. Jenny Craig and the Diet Center, with their week's worth of astronaut food that I would eat in an evening, and then starve all week. I was introduced to Prozac in my first hospital-sponsored liquid diet. It was fairly new in 1990, the appetite suppressant miracle drug, a blessing to a depressive but with absolutely no effect on my appetite. The second hospital diet introduced me to fen-phen, and it was the wonder drug it claimed to be. I could walk the streets and feel my food-antenna alert, tracking the odors—hot oil from the Chinese place, garlic from that Italian restaurant, the gust of coffee from Starbucks— but it was the twist of an addict's habit, with no stimulation attached. Fen-phen got me down to 270 pounds, but I had thirty-eight years of cryonic existence, sealed alive in fat, behind me. Fen-phen did not make me easy in my body. It merely turned off a compulsion.

Dennis couldn't turn off his drinking or his judgments; I couldn't pretend to see myself as other than enormous, cur- tailed, lonely, exiled. I had a decision to make. Settle in as best I could with my judgments of him, the rest of Trollope's novels, and a steady supply of Hostess, or become the woman wearing the man's Carhartt jacket in a chilly sunset, ready for any river I decided to joust.

I fumed as I watched a daylong *Daria* festival on MTV, hosted by none other than Janeane Garofalo, as mordant and wry as I needed her to be. As I was getting it together to ven- ture out to the bank, it finally exploded. *How dare he speak for me and* my *problems—he's nothing but a* drunk!

I can only describe the next moment by saying the ceiling talked back. I heard a retort, but not from my brain. It came from outside of myself, hovering, watching.

And you are—? The ceiling asked me to fill in the blank.

I stopped in my tracks.

I am . . .

I am exactly the same.

I can't stop eating.

My coat was on, my paycheck and Citibank card were in my

pocket, but I came to a dead halt. I crawled over my chair, fumbled for the Yellow Pages, began looking up whatever I could find on diets, eating disorders, weight loss. The number I called had a long list of meetings, starting Monday, in Staten Island and the Bronx, making it highly unlikely, I breathed with relief or regret, that I would be joining a twelve-step program anytime soon. The recording got to Saturday. There was a meeting at a church on Henry Street, in my neighborhood. I'd never seen that church, I was sure of it, but I scribbled the address and left. The church was half a block from the grocery stores D'Agostino's and Gristide's. I'd passed it millions of times, one street from my front door.

I had no excuses left. Raised on stories of Catherine of Siena and St. Teresa of Avila, I don't ignore talking ceilings. Having read Jung and Shakespeare, I don't ignore the truth.

4

DEPARTURE FROM
THE PLANET OF FAT

I knew I would go to that meeting as surely as I knew I would buy and eat any number of Entenmann's apple strudels in the next two weeks. I had to harden my resolve because I wouldn't be able to make it that coming Saturday. My friend Joan was going to be in town for the day and we had tickets to see *The Sound of Music*. Strudel was on my mind.

"Let's get a sandwich," Joan said when I met her bus at Radio City. We caught up on mutual friends and hearsay as we walked over to Broadway. I was impatient to tell her about my decision to enter a twelve-step program, but I wanted to wait until we were sitting down and I had food to absorb some of the storminess I was lugging behind me.

"Oh, that," Joan sniffed over her mile-high Carnegie Deli pastrami. "I went to one or two of those meetings. Years ago. They're all crazy in there. I couldn't take it—a bunch of fat whiners."

Maybe. Joan and I were sitting in a prematinee crowd of day-bus tourists, two overweight women among many other overweight people, gleefully gorging ourselves fatter yet on fat sandwiches and fat-clouded matzo soup. Jolliness abounded in the food free-for-all. I loved it, but that day I loved it like the Last Supper.

I bit into a dill pickle with a loud snap and considered Joan's fat whiners versus the fat celebrants we were surrounded by. The diners were joyous in their anticipation of cheesecake and *Phantom of the Opera*, many of them wearing tokens of their last excursion to Manhattan, sweatshirts announcing what play they'd seen or restaurant they'd gleefully pigged out in. I had a sudden urge to make it widely known that I wasn't one of them.

"So do you think this *Sound of Music* will finally show Maria and the Mother Superior in a lesbian clutch?" I asked Joan a little too loudly. Two Massapequa moms (we knew this because they had "Massapequa Devils" letter jackets draped on their chairs) looked at me suspiciously and ducked back into their brisket and mashed potatoes.

Joan grinned. "Not with Debbie Boone playing Maria."

"I've always wondered about the Boone family," I said. "Where do they buy their teeth?"

Had the third bite of chocolate cake pushed my blood sugar over the edge? Like Dennis, I was "turning," my viciousness a convenient disguise for my irritation—at Dennis, myself, Joan's dismissal—but especially at the crowd of Hard Rock shirts that tugged over ample midsections. Observed from the takeout counter, I would be seen as one fat body among others. It didn't matter that I was dressed in black, that I was talking smut, that an Iris Murdoch novel poked out of my bag.

Twenty years older than I, Joan was plump and drab as a

turnip. She would have said she didn't care and I would have believed her. Voted half of The Cutest Couple in her senior class half a century earlier, Joan had had her turn at being thin and found it didn't get her anywhere, although I believed she missed riding her bike on the country roads of upstate New York. Joan had "settled." She had her interesting and charming children, intellectual and artistic friends. She tried not to regret her own intellectual and artistic talents that she'd given up on.

As I steeled myself for the next Saturday, I pondered the types of women I might meet and what kind of fat lady I was among them.

There are very few social roles fat women truly occupy.

There is the lucky fat woman, the Zaftig: almost unaware of the restrictions of roles, almost innocent. There is sensuality in her obesity, a languorous participation in all things of the flesh. She tends to make excellent bread, has deep-red velvet chairs in her parlor; her clothes smell of cloves and share Georgia O'Keeffe's palette. She is jolly and has flocks of friends; her lover adores her. She always has a lover.

Definitely not me: I'd cut a path strewn with broken friendships and I had a suspicious contempt for men who like fat women. I can't keep houseplants alive.

There is the Perfectionist, polished and presentable except for this one thing: an extra 150 pounds. The Perfectionist employs eye-diverting chunky jewelry and expensive makeup and upscale fat clothes that never go out of style because they are never in style. When they are candid, Perfectionists often say that while the outside looks good—they are essential to the functioning of their offices, family, homes, and friends—their insides are a mess, eating as a reward for keeping the presentation as happy looking as possible.

I did not claim membership among them. That my obesity matched how I felt about myself was never a secret. To anyone.

There is the rather truculent so-what moxie of the Trundler, steaming along like the Little Red Engine That Could, the personification of the attitude that no one can stop her from doing what she wants (jouncing sweatily at tennis, fleshily absorbing the sun at the beach, eating con brio two orders of eggs Benedict because she is fueling her attack on life).

I was not one of them. They annoyed me, so much jiggle, so much overt indulgence, so much activity and attention-calling. *Don't they ever get a gander at themselves*, I wondered. They throttled life; I treated it as a rearguard guerrilla battle of attrition.

There is the best friend and confidante, Henry James's *Ficelle*, the intermediary between the romantic ideal of the thin, charmed, and beautiful, and of the longings of ordinary folks to approach that altar, of whom James says, "She is the reader's friend." She tends to be the secretary of groups, particularly in high school, particularly in school-spirit organizations. She will bake more brownies and wash more cars than anyone else in the effort to raise money for new cheerleading uniforms.

I was not of them. At sixteen I could see that these girls would become kindergarten teachers and secretaries, selflessly raising money for new monkey bars or bringing the same brownies in for the lawyers. I resolved never to learn to type. In truth, I wouldn't have been allowed to be a *Ficelle*. I was too noisy and iconoclastic; I made the heroes and heroines uncomfortable. Sooner or later, I made ruthless fun of them all, *Ficelles* and romantic heroines alike.

There is the dreary Orphan, without affect or direction, seen mostly in grocery stores: stretch pants, T-shirt, sneakers that splay across sockless mottled feet.

I was not one of them. They scare the shit out of me.

The Orphan's and *Ficelle*'s cousin is the Drab, who often teeters on the cusp of morbid obesity. She is neither ambitious enough to lose the weight nor committed enough to go for the coronary. If the Orphan doesn't have the heart to go to the theater, and the *Ficelle* is perkily delighted to hand out props or fill the chorus, the Drab is a permanent member of the audience. In her olive green, beige, or rusty black, she watches from the dark, indistinguishable from the crowd.

I despised her for her passivity. She makes waiting an art form, waiting for imagination and obesity to happen *to* her. Even the Orphan participates in that one thing, the drama of eating.

There is the Queen Bee, the woman who becomes obese after having been one of the charmed and beautiful, and who must now be served as well as adored by her court, so decrepit is her body and enfeebled her energy to take care of herself. At some threshold, often childbirth, she finds herself helpless against the growth of her body, then finds herself helpless in using her body. Think of Lady Alabaster in *Angels and Insects* here, the quintessential portrayal. My boss, Barbara, was one of these.

I was not one of them and I wanted, badly, to shake them.

There is the Careerist, whose eating is the metronome of her success and whose girth is a kind of proof of it, authoritative and unassailable. I rather envied her but she, too, tends to belong to the fat women among us who once passed for thin. I didn't have that baseline experience or confidence to operate from, the ability to say, "When I was young and used to care about [men/clothes/the beach]."

There is the Fag Hag, whoring herself to one gay man in particular but able to shine in a crowd of them where her gender and pulchritude become either a desexed doll or a commemoration to Judy, Bette, and Joan.

Here I excelled, taking down all pretenders. A guiding principle of fag haggery is that no Fag Hag likes another Fag Hag, possession of the unpossessable being nine-tenths of the law. Naturally I disliked Fag Hags, but fat ones were especially horrible, unworthy of the attention they got. I, on the other hand, had quite the cache of Judy Garland and Bette Davis, as well as considered critiques of their filmography, to slap down as proof of my top-flight Fag Hag claim. As well, I was a good dancer and still listened to Bronski Beat. I failed insofar as I loathed disco, but I compensated by owning a set of pink flamingo coffee mugs.

Alas, one cannot be a Fag Hag all the time. That's a Saturday night role. It was an occasional part I played, when my homosexual men had time for me.

What would they be like, Joan's whiners? I worried they would all be fat and I worried they would all be thin or a laughable ten pounds overweight. I worried at too much talk of God and AA-based platitudes.

I brushed my teeth and clipped my hair back, as much as I could fix myself up on a rainy March Saturday morning. "It'll have to do," I said as I scooped up my keys and looked around my apartment for a reason to stay home. My stomach was tense, but I couldn't say with what.

I hoped I would find the meeting without having to ask where it was, without giving myself away as one of *those people*. I hoped I would not feel as freakishly fat as I had in other weight-loss programs. I hoped it would not be an hour of crying and neuroses.

Perhaps I was hoping for hope.

Parish halls come in two colors, institutional green and institutional pink. This one was green. I slouched in, head down, and slid into the wooden chair nearest the door. A dozen normal-looking women were talking calmly about how they limited their food. They looked neither happy nor sad, as though this meeting was as much a part of their lives as going to the dry cleaners. Nor did they seem surprised at my presence, nor even to notice me at all, giving me the timorous courage I needed to look, in cautious peeps, at the group. The leader had a faded Eastern European accent and looked waifish, but she spoke with gentle assurance as she passed a stapled sheaf of papers to a pudgy, redheaded dwarf. "Will you start with the first tool?" she asked, and the woman began to read about having a plan of eating. She finished with the reading's promise of physical recovery, which caused me some worry—she was not thin—then declared herself a "food addict" and began talking about her diet.

"I don't weigh and measure, but I only eat one plate at each meal," she said.

H'mm, I thought. *How big a plate?* I thought of the brouhahas New York occasionally gets into over building high-rises on top of historical buildings or that will cast a shadow into Central Park. *Can one plate include air space?* A bubble of nerve-mirth tickled my larynx as I imagined a plate heaped like apartments on the Guggenheim, a teetering skyscraper of fried chicken, potatoes, corn, biscuits, all the way down to cake. The reader went on to say she'd gotten off of insulin after six years and that her blood pressure was now normal. My postmodern Hansel and Gretel riff came to an end as I removed the cake from my museum of overeating.

Another voice, a Heather, took up the thread from there, saying that she eschewed sugar and flour and that she weighed and measured her meals. *Oh no,* I groaned to myself. *I don't wanna*—"I've maintained a ninety-pound weight loss for three years," this Heather went on, and my eyes jerked up. Heather was ten years younger than I, with a mane of black curls, creamy skin, happy black eyes. How could she ever have weighed ninety pounds more? She was adorable. I couldn't picture how this young woman in jeans and a camisole that hovered over her flat belly button would have looked three years ago.

Numbers and achievements were being shared. Forty pounds from a gruff Brooklyn accent and Talia Shire's face. Eighty pounds from a kittenish face and serious voice. A dream backpacking vacation in the Dolomites after losing 110 pounds from a woman whose hippie-elf clothes looked so native to her that I could not imagine what she could have found to wear at 300 pounds.

Heather spoke up again with a story of cramming a package of Chips Ahoy into her mouth in the space of time it took to pee at her boyfriend's house, of brushing off the crumbs and sucking her teeth clean as she returned to his bed. Everyone roared. I roared.

And then I began to cry.

No one was surprised although they glanced at me with calm smiles that I searched for condescension or derision or robotic recruitment. I came up bumpus on meaning behind the smiles, except for a certain warmth in the eyes, and recognition as they absorbed the pleading—*tell me how to stop, how to be thin*—I embodied. The voices moved on to other topics—a woman in leather pants described eating herself out of her acting career and marriage, a latte-voice stated that she honored other people's anonymity in meetings by not advising or touching them when they were in pain—and I cried harder. Mostly thin, some chubby, one grossly overweight but on a diet at last—these women *got* it, had done it all. Eaten, been fat, lost their lives, come into a church basement and admitted the problem.

I sat with an empty chair on each side of me so that my spillage wouldn't touch, wouldn't *infect,* anyone, acutely aware that I was dressed as an Orphan: elastic-waisted pants in Lane Bryant's largest size, a black T-shirt permanently stiff with perspiration under the arms, crummy Keds, no socks, an unlined raincoat. It was 28 degrees outside and I was comfortably warm. As they talked about what had pushed them into this church, I knew that I was an Orphan and that these women knew more about me than I did.

I cried the second week, too. With my head mostly bowed, I saw the great circle of feet. And one great pair of shoes—beige Hush Puppies. Curiosity got the better of me. I lifted my eyes to the owner's face. Beautiful. Really beautiful. Blond, Michelle Pfeiffer beautiful.

That week, a thin, handsome man talked of stopping in bodegas after the sex clubs closed each weekend, gobbling Twinkies and Little Debbies in the first light of day, only to puke it all up when he got home. "I'm a binger, food and sex together," he said. "One feeds the other."

Michelle Pfeiffer spoke next. "I so relate to that. My boyfriend loves my body—why can't I? I lost a hundred pounds seven years ago and I still hate parts of my body. I'm so sick of this shit, you know?"

My head jerked up. Michele Pfeiffer didn't like the way she looked? She'd lost a hundred pounds? She'd said *shit*?

This was getting interesting.

To my surprise, Hush Puppy approached me at the break and introduced herself. "I'm Katie. I know you're a newcomer. Do you have any questions?"

For the fortieth time I broke into tears. "I don't know what to eat today."

Katie paused, sizing me up. "Why don't you call me later and we can talk about that?"

Looking back on that exchange, Katie said it was like talking to someone with her arm twisted behind her back, crying "Uncle!"

I went home and ate a box of macaroni and cheese that I'd already bought. I sorted a fat manila envelope of receipts and tallied up my expenses for that year's taxes. I looked at the phone. My underarms were clammy and my hands shook. I'd been to five meetings and had heard about sponsorship. This program seemed to be fueled on the say-so of sponsors. People referred to them constantly, saying things like "I turn my food over to my sponsor each day and then I don't have to think about it again." Not think about food? Laughable! "My sponsor suggested I take notes during my annual review. 'Don't react,' she said. 'Listen.'" Work without blubbering or justification? What planet were these women from?

Mine. The Planet of Fat. Sponsors were teaching them how to pass for human. I needed such a teacher, as well.

I'd heard the sentence, "Look for someone who has what you want and you ask that person how she or he is achieving it." At four o'clock, I picked up the phone and dialed Katie's number. She was in the middle of steaming potatoes for the week and told me it was a good time to talk.

"I love potatoes," I said.

"Me, too," she answered. "I love all my food."

I took that in. "So this abstinence thing," I asked hesitantly, "it's not about being indifferent to food?"

She laughed merrily. "How could it be? I'm an addict. I love food more than anything. It might as well be *good* food!" She went on to tell me more about how much energy she had eating the way she did, how she didn't spend time wondering what to eat, how clean she felt eating basic whole foods, what it was like to have the same clothes fit season after season. I listened. Then, with great hesitancy, I hemmed and hawed my way into "the question."

"I know you're probably really busy, and you don't have to answer right away. You can think about it. You don't have to say anything now and you don't have to say yes, I-know-you-don't-have-time-but-would-you-consider-sponsoring-me?"

A long silence. My underarms passed from clammy to wet.

"I think I have to say yes on this one," she responded.

Look for someone who has what you want and ask that person how she or he is achieving it.

I wanted to be thin. I wanted to be pretty. I wanted her shoes.

The deal was that I would have to work her program, since she would only sponsor what she herself was doing. Three meetings a week, three phone calls a day. Check, check. Oh, and I would call her every morning and tell her what I would eat that day, three weighed and measured meals with nothing in between, no sugar and no flour. Specific amounts of protein, oil, vegetables; one fruit and one carbohydrate at breakfast.

No one knows where this food plan comes from, nor is it requisite in the Rooms, the term twelve-step programs use for their church basements, community centers, and hospital conference rooms. Katie got it from her sponsor, Bridget. Bridget got it from her sponsor in another city, who got it from her sponsor, back, we hypothesize, to Moses.

"Do you want to start now or tomorrow?" Katie asked.

I had a pineapple cheese Danish in the house. Tomorrow. I wrote down the measurements, and made a list of groceries. For dinner I ate a box of Hamburger Helper lasagna with lots of mozzarella, a loaf of garlic bread, half a bottle of red wine, and most of the Danish. At four the next morning I woke in a panic, not from what I'd eaten the night before but about what I'd have to eat from now on. "What," I wailed when I called Katie at seven, "am I going to do with my madeleine pans? I can't not eat sugar and flour for the rest of my life!"

"Can you do it today?" she asked calmly.

"Yes, of course, but—"

"Then do it today."

Uncle.

I felt like an idiot as I began making a sixteen-ounce salad for lunch, first in a soup bowl, moving up through mixing bowls to the largest. I felt like a junkie as I darted out for yet more romaine, each time to a different store because of what they would think at my third visit for a head of lettuce. I felt like an incontinent child when diarrhea set in a few days later from the forty ounces of vegetables I was eating each day in place of bowel-packing starches. I felt like a dork each time day counts were called for at meetings and I was still in double digits.

In my fourth week I was standing in my kitchen, ready to make a call to Fascati's for delivery. I shook my fist at the ceiling that had started it all and demanded, "Get *down* here.

Maybe you didn't mean for me to be born, but I was, so you'd better *fucking* well get down here and do your job for a change." It was the first time I'd prayed in earnest in years. I tell my fellow skeptics to follow my food plan and I guarantee they'll get a "spiritual program." It's just too damn hard not to enlist divine help.

For all the scrambling for lettuce and worry about business lunches and the gut-twists of digestion, I felt good. Ten days after I began, I commented to my father that my twelve-Motrin-a-day habit for niggling headaches had dwindled away. "You have a food allergy," he said bluntly, echoing how food addicts refer to the compulsion-inducing toxicity of flour and sugar. "Keep doing this."

A month later, about the time the Fascati delivery man called out to me on the street, "Why I no see you anymore?" I asked Katie if she could see the eighteen pounds I'd lost. "Not really," she said. "It's more like your face has popped into focus." I was disappointed but quickly reconsidered. Focus was good. One of the things I knew going in was that the only way I could confront my three hundred–plus pounds was with a sane way to live with the loss of food. In earlier diets, I'd been unable to concentrate on much besides not eating and computer games. Perhaps this explains why I'd gone on past diets when I was in love: it gave me motivation and another fantasy besides food to lose myself in. This time I wasn't in love. If I was going to take off the weight, I would have to do my life. I had to go to the office, teach, read, clean my apartment, go to movies, and *get going*. I didn't know where, but I was restless.

Part of staying in my real life meant getting a life in lieu of eating. Twelve-step plans have lots of suggestions, and Katie required that I call people from the meetings. I hated it, but I found people with whom I didn't mind making regular check-ins. This was how I got to know Nora. I fell into her voice, plangent and silken. I could have sworn I'd known that voice in a previous life. Nora had parsed her weight loss in detail. Be-

cause I only weighed once a month, I had thirty days to find rewards beyond the scale. Nora tutored me in noticing my changing body.

"Are your shoes loose?" she asked twenty pounds along.
"My shoes and my watch were the first things to get big on
me." Sure enough, I noticed, my watch no longer left an impression in my wrist. By May, the shoes that had squinched my
toes were nearly comfortable.

"Have you rolled over on your stomach in bed yet?" she
asked as eagerly as a doting grandmother of her first grand-
child. "Does your tailbone hurt?"

These were the first changes I could marvel at. That I noticed
them quickly and that I marveled with someone who didn't
think them inconsequential or appalling was the relief of sur-
facing for air after diving for pennies.

Part of staying in my real life came from going to meetings.
It's often said the the greatest service to the Rooms is staying
abstinent, but more than once I was scared straight by someone
else's binge. I have been reassured by these stories, taking comfort in not being the only fucked-up weakling. Sometimes I've
been jealous, wanting but not daring to head to the bakery. Curiosity kept me going back. I wanted to hear the continuation
of various miniseries: boyfriends, how someone managed to
reestablish his abstinence, job interviews, biopsies, what someone looked like as she lost weight. My life was dull by comparison and I couldn't define what my miniseries was. Katie told
me to put my hand up in meetings and I gawped the first time
I was called on, searching frantically for something to fill up my
three minutes. "I ate dinner after the movies last night," I heard
myself saying. "I spilled my peas all over the floor. It was too
late to go out for more but I'd told my sponsor I'd eat peas so
I picked them all up and ate them. It was an abstinent dinner
but it wasn't clean." People laughed and I made my impression
in the wider context of the circle.

As my face became familiar and my shares lasted more than

thirty seconds, people began to respond to what I had to say. Katie's sponsor, Bridget, was my grandsponsor. Questions like whether I could take Communion went up the chain of command to her and, if necessary, to her sponsor. She gave advice, instructions, and observations when she saw a need for them. Bridget had lost 160 pounds ten years earlier and she had X-ray perceptions of me, eked from her decade's autopsy of her own compulsions and aftermaths. Cool, prone to bluntness, she terrified me, but her lack of bullshit meant her compliments and admonitions were equally trustworthy.

"Look someone, anyone, in the eye when you share in a meeting," she instructed. I balked. "Look around. No more closing your eyes and bowing your head. And *smile*." She laughed at the expression I pulled. "I know, I know. My sponsor made me do it, too. God, I hate smiling."

And then it was all right. Bridget had had to do it, too. She understood the risks—that someone wouldn't smile back, or that they would; that someone might take it as an invitation to introduce herself or call me or ask me out for coffee. These were elemental risks, the oxygen of becoming normal, of being human.

Luckily there were other women within the family that Bridget was the matriarch of. Seven of us followed the same rigorous food plan; I called us the Stepford Wives, eating in sync. It was the Stepfords' eyes I first dared to look into while announcing the triumph of having, just now, bent over to tie my shoe. Whoa! Check it out—*bent over*. I didn't have to find a ledge or a fire hydrant. I just—*bent over*. This meant I could now—here's a bit of humanity I'd never thought about—tie my shoes any time, any place.

It wasn't something I'd tell Dennis or Drake, or even some of these women who had never been as overweight as I still was. But I could look at Tracy, Bridget's other sponsee and my auntie-sponsor, smile my thrilled discovery at her, and see her dawning thrill of what we were doing mirrored back.

In turn, Tracy used me, staring me down while recounting

the experience of being called from her nurse's station to another floor—*get Tracy, she's fat, too*—to talk to a 550-pound
woman who was on a respirator because she was crushing her
own heart and lungs. "The doctors wanted me to convince her
to go into rehab. Not an eating disorders rehab but one for cardiac patients. She had bedsores the size of coasters and they had
to get three big orderlies in to turn her. She was crying in pain.
And the nurses and the doctor are looking at me and all I could
say to her was, 'This is *not* your fault. You have a disease that
makes you overeat. This is *not* your fault.' "

I let her drill me with her gaze while she talked but when she
was done, I put my head in my hands and cried. For the
woman, for myself. That's when it really hit me. My eating was
as intrinsic as the color of my eyes, as possible to cure as
epilepsy. I had a disease I couldn't cure and a thousand symptoms, including obesity, associated with it. I could wrestle with
the symptoms but I would always have to take the medicine of
the Rooms and my food plan. But it was not my fault. It wasn't
anyone's fault.

But it was my responsibility.

Those three minutes of Tracy's workweek were the beginning
of an intimate if unobligated friendship. We didn't speak every
day or know each other's last names or birth dates, but by allowing her to look me in the eye, I'd given her the driftwood
that floated her across the turbulence of revelation. By forcing
herself to look me in the eye, she had given me a fundamental
and physiological understanding of myself that absolved me of
four decades of guilt.

Tracy and I were risking visibility, whether it was in our
emerging bones or humiliations or ancient grief. We were getting the same lectures on putting our hands up to speak, on the
lack of shame in crying, on looking around and smiling. Much
as we hated it, we knew that one Saturday ten years ago, Bridget had been commanded to walk into a room and pretend to
be friendly. We could do it for one day too.

Katie and Bridget had big lives. I absorbed their mentions of plans and activities, and their gratitude that they were alive and ambulatory to do them. I had come into the Rooms to get smaller in order to get bigger—bigger out there, beyond church basements.

I was lucky in this. I already knew my heart's desires: to be thin, to publish a book with my name on it, to be sanely and mutually in love. This is the human flotsam of joy, talent, ambition, the heart. They were a long way off on March 8, 1998. I knew nothing about what was coming except that I was, a day at time, finished with wondering what to eat next. That summer I saw a woman in Heart Butte, Montana, wearing a T-shirt that read "Been there, ate that."

Amen and goodbye to all that.

5

ORBITING

One day, fifty pounds into the diet, I called Liz, an editor and friend, and asked what was new. There was a short silence; I could feel her debating an answer.

"Frances, I have to tell you: I've lost seventy-five pounds." Her tone was thrilled and apologetic, and I could feel her taking the measure of my reaction in the silence. Usually I avoided fat people, not wanting to be defined by them. I wanted to be associated with thin, pretty people—I wanted their beauty to rub off on me. I reacted to fat people like two positive lodes of a magnet, repelled to the opposite side of the room.

Liz, however, was one of those overweight women who got, without saying it, the whole psychodynamic of mutual obesity.

We would meet for lunch and order whatever we wanted. Three courses of comfort food: starters of fried mozzarella, meaty entrees with mashed potatoes, dessert. Restaurant dining with a fellow fat person was usually a game of chicken, each gauging how far the other intended to go: *What looks good to you? I hear the fish here is wonderful.* Liz and I had no congress with such insouciant nonsense, the I-don't-know-how-I-got-this-way shrug two fat people give each other warily as they order the grilled salmon while praying the busboy will place a bread basket on the table rather than offering it a slice at a time. Warmed by the rich food and our ease in eating it in front of each other, Liz and I would wreak havoc on mutual acquaintances and writers, our best vituperations fomenting gales of laughter that might—maybe—be the envy of the other diners: They're *having a good time* . . .

She was telling me, in that pause, that she'd quit our little club, that she was ceasing to be like me, that there was room in her regard for me but not as a twin sister. Thank God I could respond with my own loss.

"Isn't it *cool*?" she breathed into the phone, able now to vent her excitement.

"You mean, like every day, all day, has a *purpose*?"

"Yes," she hissed. "Even the worst day has an at-least clause written into it."

"And every time you step on the scale—"

"You get good news!"

"What do you like best?" I asked.

"Sitting on the subway. I can sit down on the subway."

"Oh, yeah," I sighed. "And finding things. Last night I found something. It was either a hip, or a tumor, I'm not sure which."

"You know, nobody really gets this."

"I wonder if it's like childbirth pain," I said. "Whether you forget about finding things and riding the subway."

"I dunno. But I can tell you this, girlfriend, I wanna find out."

.   .   .

Fifty pounds and counting, always counting, although to what end I didn't know. Dieting is a numbers game: if I lost twelve pounds a month, in six weeks I'd weigh x, and by Halloween I'd weigh y, but by the time I got to y, I'd already be chasing z. I counted days of abstinence, but not calories or grams of fat. I ate whole-milk yogurt, red meat, salad dressing made with real oil. It was much later that I examined fat and calorie contents. Nor did I exercise. My one concession was to take subways rather than cabs.

The kabala of numbers dominates dieting, but for those of us who have never been in a normal body, the numbers themselves are mysteries. Nora, my tutor in noticing and celebrating the small physical changes, had read somewhere that Jacqueline Onassis had weighed 138 pounds. Jacqueline Onassis was very tall, so surely 138 was an attainable goal? I fixated for a while on Playboy bunnies. The centerfold data said they were six feet two inches tall and 120 pounds. A good 20 pounds of that had to be in their breasts alone. Were they lying? Would I be a failure if I didn't get to 120? Rumors on the diet beat are rife. The insurance charts over- or underestimate; it's healthier to weigh ten pounds more, or less, than they recommend. At five feet eight inches, my weight, according to the Metropolitan Life Insurance Company, has a twenty-one-pound range. Was I large framed? Who knew? I'd never seen my own bones.

Nor are doctors particularly helpful. They have so little expectation of seeing obese patients lose and maintain weight that their criteria is wearily modified to settling for a healthy blood pressure.

Another myth of losing weight is that the dieter replaces her wardrobe with each size lost. I lost twelve sizes. No one has that much money, or time, for shopping, and I had enough clothes from other weight losses that for a long time I didn't need to. When, finally, I could pluck a dress and draw it away from my torso to trampoline lengths, I went to Macy's women's department, a risk because their plus sizes top out at 24. I tried on a top and was tearily relieved that the buttons didn't gap. The clerk was impatient, however. She pulled at the sleeves and said, "The shoulder pads should sit on the shoulders, not on your arms." I wanted concealment at the cost of truth, and the truth was that I was diminishing but I was also emerging.

A year and 130 pounds later, I had to buy clothes for a trip to Italy. That was how I discovered I had dropped out of the 20s, and that's when my body and the sizes it fit became points of comparison other women wanted to take part in.

Size 18 was a threshold, the size I'd managed for about ten minutes when I was a high school sophomore, twenty-seven years earlier. Would this also be a matter of a few weeks? The number was loaded, having the feel of my seventh-grade birthday. I was a *teen*, with all the skittish wooziness the word contains.

My mother's reaction to my mounting weight loss, in a Sunday afternoon phone call, unbalanced me further. "That's enough," she said when I told her about my new trousers. "You're tall. An 18 is fine for you." I argued back. An 18 is still a plus size—I was still fat. Tall women wear 4s all the time . . .

When I told Katie about the conversation, she said, "Don't talk about your size with people who've known you a long time." She was right, but the advice hurt my feelings as much as Mom's response. It was a big moment, those pants I could tuck shirts into. I wanted rejoicing and praise, and instead I was hearing ambivalence and more instructions to keep my mouth shut. Hadn't I kept my mouth shut for over a year? "No" to bread and "no" to desserts and "no" to milk in my coffee. Now I had to say "no" to talking to my mother?

Mother's next response in that phone call was just as telling: "Gee, I better get busy. You're almost as thin as I am." Not only was I breaking some definition of what *I* was, but I was putting her identity at risk as well. Part of the dynamic between my mother and me, I realized, was that I would always be fatter than she. My bachelorette pulchritude kept me the baby of the family, despite living twenty-eight hundred miles away, and it allowed her to be a little fatter than perhaps she wanted to admit. At least, she could say to herself, she was smaller than Francie.

A few months later I wore a new dress to work that showed "my figure," a euphemism I'd never thought would apply to me. Barbara, trying hard to approve of the changes, commented that it was a lovely dress but it was time for me to stop.

I rose to the bait. "It's a 14," I defended. "I have a ways to go."

"No," she said. "You're getting too small."

This was absurd. I was surrounded in that office by other women who were much smaller than I. But part of Barbara's identification of them was "thin"—just as Catherine was a Philadelphian and Beth was "married" and Rachel was a "mother." Frances was "fat." As I circled in on "thin" I was changing the status quo.

What was bizarre about my changing looks was that for once I didn't intend to put people on their guard. I was trying to pass for a rational professional even though I had, in my own mind, turned into the Count from *Sesame Street,* adding, subtracting, positing numbers of everything from street signs to myself.

· · ·

Beyond the numbers were the little rewards. I would suddenly realize I was doing something absolutely revolutionary: wrapping a bath towel around myself and tucking it securely. I cried the first time I didn't have to ask for a seat belt extension on an airplane. I cried again when I delicately lowered the tray at *my* seat.

How had my face gotten so *long*? I wondered for a couple of werewolf weeks. This business of shapeshifting had the magical mislogic of Merlin. I was living backward in time, growing smaller, with an infant's fascination with her own body. I was happy a lot of the time. I remarked to a Stepford friend that I hadn't worn my grizzly bear paw earrings for a while. Those totems had announced, to myself at least, that I would take no prisoners in the day to come, I would not be an emotional gas pump. Life was simpler on a diet. Quotidian annoyances were submerged in my overriding purpose. If I had a tough encounter with a client or broke a bottle of lotion on the bathroom floor, I bounced back with the at-least clause: *Hey, at least you're losing weight today*. It was the first raison d'être I'd had in years, as energizing as having a desperate crush except that my purpose was measured and revealed rather than carefully hidden. I had no idea that the discovery of the body I wanted to find was also the loss of the Frances I had been for forty-two years.

Having choices would mean making exclusions, not something a glutton is good at. As I took up less space I became more visible. I was not being dismissed or categorized, I was being evaluated. One person might like my smile and so attend better to the way I was describing a novel; someone else might think I was too tall and find me intimidating. My visibility would lead to evaluations of the me I could not blame on being fat.

· · ·

That April, thirteen months and 151 pounds lost, I was preparing for a business trip to Italy. I was nervous about the tempta-
tions but Bridget, a seasoned traveler, was reassuring.

"It's the Mediterranean. They invented salad. You'll have a
wonderful time. Buy shoes!"

"Shoes?" I asked incredulously. "I order mine. Wide sizes are
hard to come by."

She touched her hand to my cheek, a singular gesture. "You'd
be surprised at what fits, at how much you've changed."

"I know I've changed. I bought a size 14 dress for this trip.
A 14. Can you believe it?"

"M'mm." Her voice was neutral. "You still need to take a
good look at yourself, not just the new dress. You're lovely, you
know."

If I were a dog, I'd have been on my back, wriggling madly
from the tummy rub of Bridget's compliment.

I was so pleased I didn't consider whether I believed her or not.

I took an extra week beyond the book fair I was attending, a
blissfully quiet seven days in which I had no one to please or impress. I decided I didn't want to loiter in museums. I had a body
that wanted to walk and walk and walk. I got lost in Venice and
took whatever *vaporetto* offered itself, ending up on islands and
neighborhoods I'd had no intention of visiting.

It was a little space of time to get to know this Frances-in-
transition, taking things as they came. The first morning I
headed toward San Marco in the pearly early light of April. I
stopped to study stationery in a shop window and was struck
by the tall woman who had also paused to peruse. She had dark
hair scooped behind her ears, an air of mild, wide approbation,
and really, I marveled, terrific legs.

It was my own reflection.

I looked so rarely at the whole of myself. I shunned mirrors
when I was fat, so that the changes in my deflating body, taken
as a whole, didn't make sense to me. I was caught by surprise
when I tied the half-smile to the careless hair to the long legs. It

took a foreign country—a whim to catch the tango orchestras of San Marco before noon—to trick me out of seeing my compartmentalized self. With no one to turn to and bore with the discovery, it was mine in a way I had to slow down for. It put me on the alert. There was a *person* people were seeing, serving meals to, a person with hobbling Italian and a self-mocking sense of humor and a heart that was breaking at the very notion that it was alive in this place of Holy Week bells booming across the Giudecca and laundry whipping over canals so narrow they were nameless on the map. I could be any Frances I wanted to be.

Venice and Florence were swamped, as Easter approached, with student groups. I didn't look young among the waves of smooth, honeyed flesh. I'd heard every variation on the tastes of Italian men. They were interested only in skinny California blondes; they liked a little meat on a woman; they were mama's boys; they hated women; they were gigolos looking for a green card. In any case, it didn't matter—I was out of the sexual loop with all eyes turned on the Danish undergraduates.

And yet.

I was heading back to my hotel, my thoughts absorbed in nothing much as I rounded a corner onto the deserted *calle di scuola*. I looked up in the same instant as two young men who were unloading a boat, the three of us blinking in surprise at the appearance of each other in the lull of midafternoon. It was too sudden to look through them or off to the side, and just as quickly my eyes dropped to my feet, which I could actually see—*see*, mind you, after years of having to crane to see over my breasts and stomach and billowing hemlines.

"Hallo!" one of them said involuntarily, and all three of us grinned at the meaning, an appreciation without intent. I would be gone as soon as I appeared; they would continue unloading lumber from the boat.

But it was not idle startlement. I was less frightened by their appraisal than I was by my own. I was in my body enough to know it was my body we were all looking at.

That "hallo!" was as close to a gasp, and one of my closest encounters with feeling beautiful, as I've experienced yet.

A month later, in May, my movie life of wandering around Florence and Venice faded to a movie memory. Summer was no calendar-promise but a reality. Across the street, the Gap was mobbed with shoppers looking for shorts; in Starbucks, where the Stepfords had gathered after a meeting, they were doing a brisk business in iced coffee. A longtime Stepford, Tethys, was talking about a bash in the Hamptons she was preparing for. That morning she had tried on a dress she was pleased to announce fit for the first time. I shut my eyes in order not to wrinkle my nose. With a name like Tethys, self-chosen—Titaness, the mother of rivers—such a dress had to be sheer, floating, layers of sea colors. Tethys was one of the girliest Stepfords, definitely part of the Planet of Girls where there are parties in the Hamptons.

"The Goddess has given me a beautiful body," she purred. "I have learned to love it. I'm strong, I have curves, generous curves, that men look at. This no longer scares me. I'm beautiful and I know that the Goddess has given me this beauty along with the talent and the strength to share it. It means something, my beauty. It makes people pay attention when I sing, and my singing helps them."

She mentioned that she weighed 171 pounds.

I am two inches taller than Tethys and that day I weighed 176 pounds.

I opened my eyes, looked around to see if anyone else found it amazing that she could be on her way to a posh do at such a weight. *You'd think,* I grumbled to myself, *she'd consult an insurance chart and shut up until she hits a number it recommends.* No one else was askance and I reminded myself to have no opinion. I lowered my eyes in sardonic contemplation of my lap.

I was wearing, that prematurely hot morning, the Coney Island shorts from 162 pounds ago. *Thank goodness for drawstrings,* I'd thought earlier. They'll see me through another summer. And I liked them. Plaid flannel, soft after much wearing, their bagginess eased some of my embarrassment in wearing shorts.

Katie was sitting next to me. I'd wanted for fifteen months to be as pretty as she. She, too, was wearing shorts. My thighs were smaller than hers. She was twenty-five pounds lighter than I but my thighs were smaller.

Starbucks tilted a little. I looked at those Stepfords who, like me, were still losing weight. Erica hadn't lost a pound in a year, nor had Tracy. If someone coming in from the glare of Montague Street looked at us, I would not be clumped with Erica and Tracy. They had been my comrades-in-arms, but suddenly I was one of the—what? Fairly normal, almost thin, the slightly overweight, which included Tethys, whose confidence cowed me into ranking her queen among the Girls. In my enormous shorts with my small dull life, I had lost my tribe, my fellow emigrants from the Planet of Fat. I studied Katie and Tethys for what made them Girls. It wasn't whether they were thin. There was other stuff going on. Shiny skin and the scent of lotion and painted toenails and thought-out hair. They looked around, looked people in the eye. I didn't have a clue about how Tethys or Katie did this—this *girl thing*.

It was a personal attack on my definitions of myself. "Fat" was fading. "Thin" was minutes away, and I had only now gotten it that thin included being feminine. I was on my own. I was in free fall. I was outraged.

. . .

As I made the rounds of my neighborhood that afternoon, I studied the fat women. How they peg-walked because their thighs pushed their feet apart. How their breasts moved in counterpoint to their bellies. How they dressed in dark long-sleeved shirts and double-knit pants so snug they showed the dimples in their knees. How they kept their arms clamped at their sides. How their stomachs preceded them so that the person herself showed up a millisecond later.

I no longer moved like that. My body was all in one place, one motion. My ankles were bruised because I kept knocking my heels against them, not yet adjusted to the new center of gravity in my body. I'd changed from being one of the fat with dieting as my main occupation to a creature half alien, half human. I'd loved—truly loved—having the constructive purpose in life of lots of weight to lose, of putting off brain waves like a dream of being a Doubleday editor for "later." Later was the goal of more weight lost, an arrival I'd assumed had some kind of finish line: a *number*, a size, a date. I was incredibly sad. On the one hand I'd lost my tribe, and on the other I wasn't done. But finishing was within reach and thin was more than sighing over shorts that were too big. I'd have to actually *do something about them*, the same words I'd sighed ineffectively over my weight for forty years.

In my fifteen months in the Rooms I'd seen a lot of refusal to join the world for the manifold pleasures and possibilities a thin body offered. If femininity confused me, I was hell-bent on mastering it anyway.

The first time I heard there was a thing called an eating disorder I hooted. "I don't have an eating disorder! I order just fine—

take-out, delivery, restaurants; Italian, Chinese, Mexican. You name it, I can order it." I heard my former defiance in visiting aliens' resistance. "I don't know why I'm here," said a woman who showed up every few months. "I'm too busy for you people. I'm writing and directing films and I don't have time to sit around and talk about this. I'm fine." She was a solid two hundred pounds overweight. *Can you line up a camera angle with that gut?* I wanted to argue back. *How would it feel to have a lap to hold your toddler on?* Visiting aliens made me think what an easy body might be like, and they reinforced how powerful denial is. "It ain't just a river in Egypt," Mark Twain pointed out.

Passing as a Girl would mean emotional continence as well as table continence, a diet for my personality. *Get over it*, my mind chattered back when another hostile launched a five-act drama. I could do nothing but tune out the shrillness and apply those three words to myself: *get over it.*

Tethys with her chiffon, Katie with her sweeping gilded hair. They got to be Girls and I was in a netherworld, neither thin nor Girl nor fat, unsure until I got there what I was supposed to weigh. Twenty-four hours later I was in a full-out breakdown. I belonged nowhere, to no one. I made a rare call to Katie outside of our scheduled times. "Place your hand where it hurts," she advised, referring not to my heels or the insides of my knees and elbows that were sore without the cushion of fat. My hand splayed across my upper chest with its new topography and rested over my heart, thumping palpably under the ribs. I hugged my knees and rocked in my straight-backed chair. I hadn't been able to hug my knees since grade school.

By August 1999, I could produce some amazing numbers: 14,400 pounds of salad consumed; 1,800 ounces each of fruit, vegetables, and yogurt; 570 days of back-to-back dieting and the only flour or sugar I consumed in that time had been the Communion wafer and wine on Ash Wednesday. My top weight was 338 pounds. I weighed, that August, 168 pounds. Total loss: 170 pounds.

I was filled with nervous energy, no longer needing ten hours' sleep and finding my natural rhythm of waking at four-thirty. But I was chronically weary, a different thing from being tired, pale as clouds under a full moon. Katie had been talking about modifying my food plan to slow down my weight loss and so far I'd resisted. When I called her on July 31, she announced that she and Bridget had talked over my wan listlessness.

"It's time, Frances," she said. "You've lost weight faster than anyone I've ever sponsored, and your body's worked hard. But it's tired. We need to help it."

I could not be goal weight. I weighed more than Dennis, who is five inches taller than I. But the last time I weighed 168 pounds was in fifth grade—what did I know?

Saner people than I had gotten me to 168 pounds; I had to take their evaluation seriously. Four days before I left for a visit to Montana, Katie added a six-ounce carbohydrate to my lunch and a fruit to my dinner.

And that was that. The difference between rapidly and consistently losing weight, and maintaining it, is a six-ounce potato and one fruit. That's how narrow the pavement is.

I had a few days to adjust to the carbohydrate (yam or Idaho? steamed or baked?) and fruit (before I washed the dinner dishes or after?) before getting on a plane and facing my childhood, 145 pounds smaller than two years before. I was so identified with what I ate that a yam and a mango tipped my definition of who I was even further. Now I ate in courses, a normal occurrence for a thin person. More than one dish, a third item in restaurants. That movie Frances wandering around Murano, Tethys's glamorous perception of herself, Katie's disappointment in her thighs, my billowing shorts, the bag of rice cakes in my cupboard—these were the mosaic tiles in the carry-on baggage I would be taking to Montana.

"I can't wait to see you," Lisa gushed on the phone the night before I left, and she meant it literally. I was about to be *seen,* for the first time, as I truly looked in the flesh rather than the fat, and by people who were used to seeing other aspects—"the problem of Francie," her sarcasm, her gobbling, the waste of such a pretty face—whether I was ready or not.

6

ARRIVAL ON

THE PLANET OF GIRLS

Jim and I met the family at Applebee's, one of a dozen restaurants on Missoula's Strip—Highway 93 as it empties south into the Bitterroot Valley. There is nothing about Missoula that doesn't summon memories, but it was fitting that Mother chose a restaurant across from what were the fields I knew intimately thirty years ago and the house I grew up in. That house now belongs to someone else and I avoid looking at it, knowing they've taken out the aquariums, and reconfigured rooms. Wal-Mart has filled up the pasture that was home to a half dozen friendly horses. Jim's youngest kids would never be able to take off on their bikes in the impatient traffic, never be able to put pennies on the railroad tracks or pick wild asparagus. The old days have been reduced to replications like this restaurant, hung with washboards and wagon wheels and Gibson girls selling long-defunct brands of beers. It was meant to be nostalgic and homey. I had never felt less at home and my nostalgia was tinged with bitterness and regret at the loss of countryside, the loss of being known here, even if it had meant looking like the Pillsbury Dough Girl.

Put that family lunch after I got off the plane in Missoula into forty-two years' context and perhaps the lack of reaction I got from the small crowd of Kuffels—eleven of us, four generations—wasn't surprising. They might have been following my father's lead—he gave up flamboyant reaction sometime around Lindbergh's crossing of the Atlantic—except that he had a golf game and was the one personage missing from the table. They were as uncertain of what my reaction to them would be as theirs would be to me. I could have wagered someone had asked, "Which Francie will walk through the door?" Jim and I were known for yearlong silences after flinging my humanism in the eye of his right-wing politics and theology; except for Lisa, I barely knew my nieces and nephews at all. Francie could walk in as the jolly one, the confrontational one, the prankster, or the sullen or superior or generous or hiding one.

Behind door number three was a new and combo permutation: the edgy-balky Francie.

They had filled a big booth, with a couple of chairs drawn up to complete the circle. Nine people waved Jim over, seven of them—Justin and Sophie were too young to remember me—craning to see me behind him.

"Hi, hi," I said in a breathy voice. My lungs weren't quite working and I sounded more like my nieces than my own gravelly alto. Lisa, Brenda, and my mother jumped up. Lisa was already talking—fast, her conversation rhythm always reminded me of eating corn on the cob or a ticker tape machine—a rush of saving me a place and how was the flight and where did Jim find me. My sister-in-law, Brenda, stepped in to hug me, hard, a beat or two longer than I would have hugged her, and whispered in my ear, "It's good to see you. You look . . . *great*." By the time I got away and Mom got a quick kiss in, Lisa was pushing me onto the banquette. The ranks of my family closed around me.

There was a whole lot of looking going on, covert sips of my face, and tiny time lapses before addressing me. My youngest niece, Kim, has never been able to control her affect; expressions and feelings flit nakedly across her face. Her eyebrows were drawn together in consternation and the corners of her mouth quicked when I caught her staring, more frankly than anyone else dared to.

It was when I spoke—having gotten a couple of breaths, my voice had returned to husky, my pronunciations touched by New York speed and open vowels—that they relaxed a little and took in the rest of me.

"Great shirt, Francie," my sister-in-law, Brenda, said. "It makes your eyes so blue. I've never seen them so blue before."

Of course not, I could have answered. *They were sunk in bulge.*

"Thanks," I said instead, as Katie had instructed me.

Kim was still watching, her eyes riveted even when she turned her head to listen to a plan my grandniece, Kaylie, had in mind. Her staring was eerie. I couldn't think of an instance when someone had been so fixated on me. I took a deep breath and dived in.

"So, Kimmie, what's new?"

"Nothing."

"Something has to be new," I coaxed. "What are you doing with your summer vacation? Are you quilting with Mee-maw"—Jim's youngest kids' name for my mother—"or doing other crafts?" Kimmie sped through her days at breakneck speed, flitting from one project to another, assiduously careful in her handiwork but with the attention span of gnat.

"Not really."

So much for small talk with nine-year-old number one. I turned to Kaylie, nine months younger than Kim. "How about, you, Kay? What are you doing this summer?"

Kaylie stared at me a moment, her eyes wide, then turned to Jamie, my niece. "Mother," she whispered hoarsely. "Who *is* she?"

Jamie giggled, one of the most musical giggles in the Pacific Northwest. "That's *Francie. Francie*. Remember? She towed you around the lake in your raft?"

"*Oh, yeeaahh*. That was so much fun . . . Francie."

Kimmie's eyes had been watching this conversational ball flick back and forth. The mention of the lake gave her a chance to summon the Francie she remembered.

"Will you bake cookies with me, Francie?" she asked. All of my brothers' progeny had memories of baking with me. "Will you go swimming with me? Can we play Monopoly?"

It was all coming back to her now. I smiled. "Some of that, yeah. We'll see what happens, OK?"

She smiled, her teeth too big for her face, the nine-year-old's curse. She was still watching me but she was easier now. She was merging her history together with my face.

This has gotta be as hard on them as it is on me, I thought. Part of what was hard on all of us was how legible my face was without its indeterminate muddle of chub. Not only were they seeing what I looked like, but every expression (Mother had been trying to curb it for years, since my face always informed the world what I was feeling about it, not often peaceful) etched itself with stylus-clarity. I hoped they saw bafflement and shyness as well as the facts of features they also had to acquaint themselves with. High cheekbones and bigger, bluer eyes, my face looked its age without the collagen of obesity, lines from my nose to my mouth that turned to pleats when I smiled, lines in my forehead that turned to furrows as I read the menu.

My food may have reminded them that it was really Francie, at least in volume. It had been nine hours since breakfast and I was jittery as I ordered the lunch that approximated my requirements of vegetable, protein, and whole-grain carbohydrate. "Wow," my niece Jamie said. "That's a lot of food." Ten pairs of eyes swiveled as I ate my salad and chicken, rice and overcooked "fresh" vegetables of the day.

"This is what I'm supposed to eat."

"It's a great food plan," Lisa chimed in, on the frisky side of savage. "What is it, about six hundred calories and none of it sugar?" She shares my compulsions with food, and were it not for the hundreds of miles she runs each week she could have been me.

My grandnephew's loud insistence that he had wanted chicken fingers instead of a hamburger distracted us from that dangerous path. "The toddlers are even harder to feed than me," I joked to too-hearty laughter from the five adults. *Francie's still funny.* I smiled, but it was a small smile. A grin might have split me down the middle and my questions might come spilling out. *Am I pretty? How much bigger am I than you? Do you love me—still love me, or love me more for having done this? Did you love me before? Was it possible to love me when I was fat? What do you love now? Am I gonna be OK—be a person, be Frances? Will I figure this out? How? What have I done?*

Mother broke the tension of maintaining the same-old, same-old nonchalance. Leaving Applebee's two hours later, she reached out and swatted me across the butt.

"Your pants are too big."

"I ironed them," I said defensively. "They got creased on the plane."

"That's not what I said," she answered with a look that said *be quiet and think.*

I'd bought the khakis four months ago. My criterion for pants was based on whether I could feel the waistbands. Drawstrings and elastic afford almost no physical sensation at all, so actually feeling my clothes was a new and misleading sensation.

Because I could feel the waist of these, I assumed not only that they fit but that they were *tight*.

"They're comfortable."

"I'm sure they are," she said dryly. "And you look like a clown from behind."

They were the very trousers, in fact, the 18 to which Mom reacted that I should stop losing weight because I was "tall."

Listening to us, Lisa laughed. I had a doctor's appointment and then Mom would take me to Lisa's house to spend the night. She was collecting fodder for dishing the family and was keen to make a physical assessment of me. Lisa is the only person, familial or social, who has never, once, disapproved or lectured or shaken her head over me. Or given me up as hopeless.

This was pure celebration for her. I was glad—at least someone got to enjoy my body. I wanted my victory lap, but I had hurdles left to jump before I could slow down and wave at the crowd.

My doctor, Jesse, had been one of my father's surgery pals. Out of their mutual regard, I'd been sent to Jesse as a doctor who would understand me. Jesse did. He refrained from the disapproval I got from other doctors, appreciated me for being my father's daughter and for my accomplishments over the fifteen years I'd been going to him. This year they were booked. I'd resorted to bribery.

"Last August I asked Jesse what weight he wanted me at," I explained to Mom. "He told me he'd be happy if I got to 200 and that he'd do a handstand if I got to 180. I told his secretary that I weigh 168 pounds now and I want my handstand. I told her she could come watch." Mom grinned.

"I'm sure she was able to jiggle the schedule," she said. "There's always time for an old patient from out of town."

The scale was wrong, I informed the nurse. I weighed four pounds less.

It was the first time I'd allowed his nurse to tell me my weight, although once she muttered it under her breath and I'd nearly decked her.

Jesse's staff is loyal, they've been with him forever, and they edged closer as I went through the preliminaries. No one said anything.

"I hear Doc Kuffel's kid is in today—where is she?" The door banged open. The coming joke failed as he gawked.

"I want my handstand," I said. "I brought my mother as a witness."

"Where is she?" he asked, and stepped back into the hall. "Where's Mrs. Kuffel?" he yelled. "Someone bring her back here."

Mother came in, twinkling. Jesse twinkled right back at her. "So."

"So," she said.

"What do you think?"

"I think she's beautiful."

"She's always been beautiful."

"What does her father say?"

"He hasn't seen her yet. He's golfing."

She's always been beautiful.

I didn't get a handstand. I didn't get much of an exam or to participate in the conversation, a strange confab about me, about my father's golf game. But Jesse's third-person glee gave my mother a blueprint she would use in the coming days and the years. *Look at her—isn't she beautiful?*

Look at me. Look at her. Look at you. So much depends on grammar.

First person is scathing. It demands that I define myself. The first person presumes I have some idea of what I have changed into when all I really have is a limited accuracy of comparing myself to myself, and in the most general terms. I am smaller than I was. That's trustworthy enough. That I can feel ribs I couldn't a month ago is less trustworthy. Had I just not noticed? Is it a weight *shift,* or loss?

Questions are annoying. "How do you feel?" seems to call for answers along the lines of "light as a feather." I don't. "Pick up a twenty-pound bag of potatoes and imagine you're carrying that," I'd been told a million times in my obesity. It was a fallacy. My 170 pounds had not been in a bag or a hump on my back, it had been distributed evenly over my frame, like a suit. How do I feel? The truth? Tired, like everybody else, but the interrogator hears it as drained and anemic from dieting. "Tickled because last night I curled up in a movie seat" is too intimate, too telling of where I come from and likely to spur other questions I may not want to answer. Curiosity about the means is an invitation to argument: "You can't eat chocolate? I could never give up chocolate." "Seventeen months? That's all? Did you exercise?"

Having last been seen 100 or 140 pounds ago, at least no one asked *why* I did it.

It was in second- and third-person statements that I began to find answers about the body I inhabit. One day that summer my officemate, Catherine, paused on her way to fetch a ream of paper and remarked on my broad shoulders. My hand lifted protectively to my collarbone, invoking the gods of weight distribution. When would I lose weight *there*? It was another body part I'd never thought about. She laughed. She'd seen every pound I'd lost, knew what such gestures meant. "No, Frances. Broad shoulders are *good*. Clothes are *designed* for broad shoulders. You have the body they make clothes for."

I needed these statements and evaluations. What is called for as an antidote to the sting of doubt and instant amnesia is a surrender of self-diagnosis in favor of faith in someone else's powers of objectivity. Second and third person had to be invoked.

"Oh-Kaay," Lisa rubbed her hands together as I dropped my suitcase in her guest room. "Now I have you where I want you. I wanna see everything."

I unzipped my suitcase. "I have picture books for Sophie," I said as I started digging around. "A friend at Houghton Mifflin sent these over. They're about sharks and whales. I think she'll like them." I held out a lurid red book. "And the new Tom Harris. For you, not Sophie." I handed her the stack of books.

"Sophie hates it when you give me books. 'Mom, come *back*,' she kept saying when you sent that geisha book. I couldn't stop reading."

I bent over to flap the top of the suitcase closed from prying toddler and dog.

"Nuh-uh."

I looked up. "What?"

"What else is in there?"

"Sorry, kid. Santa's sleigh is empty."

"I want to see your new clothes."

"I don't have anything interesting," I said. "It's Montana. I didn't need to go shopping for three weeks at Flathead."

"You didn't buy anything new?"

"Only a swimsuit."

A demonic gleam seized her. She yanked the suitcase over. "Put it on."

"Why?"

"I want to see what happened to you."

It was a day of stripping off my clothes. First for Jesse, now for Lisa's burning curiosity at what I'd turned into. Only for Lisa would I take off my clothes like that. She was a veteran of the war with the scale, hitting two hundred when she was pregnant and, that summer, still nursing, settled into baggy T-shirts and no-size shorts. I could trust her on two counts: she loved me no matter what, and she had some idea of what I was dealing with.

She laughed out loud at my bra and underwear, which hung in pleats. I hadn't bought a bra in a store since I was fifteen years old, had ordered undies from Lane Bryant around the time I started losing weight. I looked at myself in undress as little as possible.

She held out my swimming suit as I more or less let my underwear fall off. My old suit had died and I'd ordered a Speedo from Lands' End, following their diagrams with a bathrobe belt, ruler, and much rescribbling on scrap paper, coming out a disappointing size 16.

"You'll have to do something about your beard," she said, and I lifted the bulge of my stomach to see that, yes, pubic hair sprang out around the edges, something I'd never dealt with in the boxy suits with skirts I'd favored before.

My cheeks burned. Pubic hair—ugh. It was so . . . messy, out of control, blatantly female. I was messy and out of control for having it.

"What do I do?"

"I shave mine," she answered. I breathed a little deeper. I wasn't the only one with the problem.

"Turn around," she went on briskly. I rotated, my stomach pooching out in the black spandex, my arms jiggling. What I really needed was a bathing *costume,* hose and bloomers and a stripy shift à la *Death in Venice.*

"Your legs are great. You always had great legs. But it's re-markable, Franny—really weird. You're so thin you're not *there.* Your body isn't where I expect it to be. You're not . . . Franny."

I lifted my stomach again, a more than generous hang, and slapped my upper arms and thighs loudly. "I'm all here. This isn't thin."

"Yeah, but it all gets covered up." She looked at my open suitcase and her nose twitched. "Let's look at your clothes. We have to go shopping. What else do you need?"

"Phoo," I exhaled. "Nothing. I went shopping in May." I thought a moment. In my suitcase were linen sacks, soon to out-seasoned. "Fall clothes, I guess. And T-shirts." There were some hilarious Montana T-shirts I'd brought back to New York as presents over the years, amusing friends with what was one of my secret shames. I didn't fit them.

"We'll do that tomorrow. What are you making for dinner? I love your salads."

Lisa bounded into my parents' house on the East Shore of Flat-head Lake, yakking a mile a minute about the drive, the lunch I'd made, Sophie's tantrum that fizzled into a long nap as soon as we left the interstate. Mother asked the questions that en-couraged more chatter; Daddy sat at the dining room table reading mail and grunting occasionally in response. Lisa switched to questions.

"Grandpa?" she said.

One eyebrow raised incuriously from the Publishers Clearing House ads.

"Grandpa, we have to figure out Francie's body."

"Two arms, two legs, one head. That's what I learned in the olden days. Have things changed?"

"No. We have to figure out what's what on it." She dragged me in front of him. "Look at her arms."

"So?"

"Feel them."

She pulled my arm out. He clasped my ulna, squeezed, let go. "Definitely attached."

"No, Grandpa. Her *upper* arm."

He took my hand and drew me closer, the clasp different— gentler, reassuring a frightened patient, but ready to probe. His fingers massaged my prodigious bicep.

"Fat," I said sadly. "It's one of my fat spots."

"Skin," he countered.

"No way. It's thick. Feel it. I still have a lot of weight to lose there."

"It's skin, honey. Skin is heavy."

"She needs to lift weights, doesn't she?" Lisa demanded.

"If you say so," Dad said, letting go and picking up another catalogue. "If you're thinking it will make the skin go away, it won't. Weights build muscle, they don't reduce skin. She'd have to be Popeye to fill that skin. But it wouldn't hurt—she's a wimp."

"Yeah, but look at her legs," she protested, ready to defend me even against my defenders. "Her legs aren't wimpy." She yanked my shorts up and he peered over the tops of his glasses at my legs, the vein that rippled from my crotch to my left knee, spider veins, the antimacassar of skin draping my knees.

"No, they're not. I'm surprised, actually. She's lost very little muscle tone in her legs." He slapped my right thigh lightly. "A little, but that's mostly skin, too." He looked up at me. "What are you going to do about that vein?"

"What can I do?" I sighed.

"Strip it. You'll have to pay unless your doctor refers you for medical reasons. I want you to go in and complain of tiredness in that leg. That should do it."

"But she has runner's legs, right?" She turned to me. "You have runner's legs."

How reassuring. Lisa has her own ideas of what a fit body can do with itself, involving miles of sweat spilled in places meant for mountain goats.

"Whatever." Dad does not cotton to middle-aged marathon sports.

She wrinkled her nose at me. "You can run. It's all right."

Swell.

"Now." She took up her mission. "Her stomach. What about her stomach?"

"I have a fat stomach," I said. "It's fat." Lisa was relentless as she tugged my shirt out of my shorts. This was asking a lot. I had a surgical scar running from stem to sternum, wrinkles and folds, stretch marks. My belly looked like Normandy from twenty thousand feet, hedgerows, canals, craters, and one big highway right through my navel.

"It's fat," he agreed. "You have a fat stomach."

I was disappointed. But this is Daddy. He always told us as kids that if we wanted sympathy, we'd find it between shit and syphilis in the dictionary.

"Also skin. You have fat and skin." He lifted the new issue of *Discover* and looked at us both. "Are we done now? I can read now, right? It's good to see you, kid."

He got up to go to his reading chair and kissed me on the nose. I took his hand in our parody of an eighteenth-century courtier's invitation to a dance. We stepped back and swayed up and in to bump tummies.

Except it was really *in*, our faces nearly touching, it was his tummy keeping us at bay. The dance we'd adopted from *Fantasia*'s "Dance of the Hours" sagged. He stepped back and shook his head. "Doesn't work like it used to. You did good, kid."

Neither my mother nor I knew Missoula's clothing stores anymore. The atelier of my mother's halcyon days as doctor's wife and career woman had long-since closed, the hippie shops of muslin and tie-dye that I'd never fit were no longer appropriate. There was a new culture in town—out-of-state money, California and New York money—supporting little dens of Tyrolean wools and hybrid sporty office wear that seemed either fussy or sentimentally prairie chic, at prices that made me, a New Yorker, used to paying three bucks for a cup of coffee, gag. Mom trolled gamely up Front Street, passing in and out of shops I was relieved to reject. She wanted to buy me something wonderful. I wanted not to have to try anything on. I didn't want any more disconcerting truths.

But we both love clothes. We were near the Kiddie Shop, the last place she'd gotten to indulge her fantasies for me. It had been a thrill standing on the soldier's drum with three mirrors reflecting my image. I vividly remember the dresses she chose, sometimes for their girliness, sometimes with a streak of precocious maturity. My dresses were characters in my days. I named them: the Omaha Dress, Shawn's Birthday Party Dress, the Cinderella Dress. I know it was one of her disappointments that she didn't get to dress up her doll-baby, a family term of affection, past first grade.

"Let's go to the Bon," she sighed. Mom is in her late seventies and sensitive to extremes of temperature; the heat was taxing her arthritis.

The Bon used to be The Missoula Mercantile, and it used to be an event to go to our one department store (white gloves and good behavior) and to lunch at the Florence Hotel across the street (a grilled tuna fish sandwich and pumpkin pie). You can tell how long Missoulians have lived there by whether they call it the Bon or the Merc. My father moved to Missoula in 1929. I still called it the Merc.

I'd have known the smell anywhere: old building, new clothes, perfume, starchy floor wax. I'd bought a peach satin bra here when I weighed 204 pounds at fifteen, and a horrible pinafore sort of shirt that was popular for the same minute I could wear it. Mom had bought me an equally horrible red car coat, the only one in town that fit, that made me look like a fire truck my freshman winter in college.

I couldn't turn around without a story or an association, and I could have told you what I ate before, after, or during.

Mother aimed straight for what they called "better clothes"—not the back-to-school clothes but the suits and dresses this booming new crop of women lawyers and brokers of inflated real estate wore.

The racks were tightly packed and overfull. I was afraid of knocking something over. I was afraid of this whole ordeal, scared I was still a 14 and we should be in the "women's department" (as if one had to be mature to be bigger than a 16, or bigger than a 16 to be mature) after all. I was scared I was smaller, scared of the mythical sizes the girls in high school talked about. Those were the girls I had wanted to be twenty-seven years ago when the smell of this place wedged itself permanently into my brain.

Mom was on the prowl, alert as a spaniel in a cornfield in pheasant season. She clacked through hangers. Swoops of material were checked and dismissed, sleeves curling around other garments as she worked her way through. It was an amazing moment, Olympian for such a tiny woman, gammer-legged in golf togs and blazing white sneakers. She had the laser-focused ferocity of an archer.

Within minutes she had zeroed in on a jacket in the scariest chartreuse God never intended, a suit that screamed "Blaine Trump has entered the building!" It was on sale, the only one, a size 8.

Mother had been a size 8 when I was in nursery school. She lived on coffee and grapefruit in order to model for Medical Auxiliary luncheons and had first dibs on the best things Cecil, the arbiter of Missoula fashion in 1961, got in. Size 8 is probably my mother's idea of the first step toward beatification. She held the label of that blazer and rubbed it between her fingers as if it were Aladdin's lamp. Thinking, imagining, pondering.

I had at least one thought in common with her: *Not possible*.

To wear it would take all the courage I possessed. I'd be worn out by that suit by 9:45 in the morning.

She rubbed. The lemon-colored lining scritched. She smoothed the blazer out across the rack of clothes, patting it, coaxing it. She looked at the price tag. She looked at me.

"Do you like it?" she breathed, and for a second I was shopping with Jackie Onassis.

"Sure," I said. Why not? It *was* beautiful. So is Mount Everest and I wasn't going near it anytime soon either. It was an 8, I was safe.

I made the mistake of listening to her voice rather than attending the expression in her eyes, which were black and hard with resolve as she rucked through a carousel of skirts and pulled out the match, a plaid chartreuse the size of a dish towel. She whipped around and held them out to me.

"I'll get us a dressing room."

She sighed in relief that the dressing room had a seat. I stripped off the linen dress I'd bought from a catalogue that June, a dress that had become a sack, hanging it up slowly. The cups of my bra were half filled and six hooks took up most of my back. She sighed again at that. I slid with effort into the skinny skirt and insinuated myself into the jacket. She stood up and starting tugging, shoehorning me into it, tamping and rearranging flesh until it zipped with an excruciating slow-motion that warned *this will not hold . . .*

She stepped back and twirled her finger for me to turn. Her brows knit with worry, approval, determination. This was emphatically *not* a case of stage motherism. It was what her thin, sophisticated, beautiful daughter deserved. I could see homage in her inspection. She was determined that suit and her daughter deserved each other.

"It's gorgeous, but it's maybe too tight?"

"Maybe," I squeaked.

"Take it off, then." Another sigh as she headed out of the dressing room and I unzipped it, one tooth at a time.

She came back with something lovely, a blue that was almost black but then flashed to teal as it caught the light, a sort of suede skirt and soft blazer, a size 10. I fell in love on the spot. "Oh God, oh God," I prayed silently, the Prayer of Special Intentions to Our Lady of Dressing Rooms. It fit. It fit beautifully. Mom smiled a smile so rare, so charmed with privilege and delight, that it was like lying in the August grass, night-watching, nearly asleep, when the Perseids break loose in one spraying flash of luck and dreams. I looked from her smile to myself in the mirror. Tall, black hair gone cranky, my eyes a bright navy blue and my complexion unsallowed from the flattering color, the blazer buttoned so that it showed my waist. This time, I said it: two words I had never, ever said out loud, stripped of "someday I think I could be," to another person.

"I'm pretty."

. . .

The suit prompted photo sessions in the backyard. A couple of years and changes of hairstyles later, they still adorn my parents' refrigerator. In looking for jewelry to go with the suit, Mother gave me the jade and moonstone sets my father brought back from Japan during the Korean War. These circlets of round stones in filigree always impress editors, but it's nothing compared to my forty years' admiration of them. The gift was the delicate admission of many things: how much Mother loved me and the ways I was turning out, the reclamation of hope she'd lost the last time we tried the Kiddie Shop and came out empty-handed. As well, she handed over this evidence of her own romantic past as a beautiful woman to another beautiful woman with her own romances ahead of her.

Someone always had a camera aimed at me that trip. I've got a million photos in my trunk but I framed the one of my father and me standing together. There's something in my face—the lines around my smile, and the newly articulated muscles in my neck—that approximates the dimples and chiseled features of my eleven Kuffel cousins. He looks incredibly happy, and I adore my father. I look, for the first time, like a Kuffel.

7

SETTLEMENT
HOUSE

New York's exhilaration in the liquid warm September on my return from Montana spilled into the streets and lazed into flirtatious nights. I weighed 168 pounds. It was the first time since March 9, 1998, that I had not lost weight. Given that I'd been on vacation, when many people gain weight, it was a triumph. The aim, now, was not each month's new set of numbers but keeping and making something out of the numbers I'd achieved. Size 10; 170 pounds lost; 590 days of continuous abstinence. Raw materials, but of *what*, exactly? Looking for answers, I took to walking and spying. A size medium, I was invisible in my normality as I prowled the clothes I might want to wear, the kinds of people I might want to belong to, glimps-

ing apartment interiors and crowds outside theaters and clubs.
I imagined myself in each of them, looking for the Eureka!
moment that would tell me about the Girl I was turning into.
The Upper East Side, Chelsea, the Village, SoHo, Brooklyn
Heights—which was mine? Or better yet, which was *me*?

Third Avenue was my work beat. I'd make a quick Starbucks
run, grab emergency tampons, pick up four ounces of roast
lamb for lunch, trace and retrace the route to the subway, shop
for birthday cards. Third Avenue had it all and I was out there
several times a day, five days a week. The restaurants in the seventies had sidewalk tables and did a brisk business as the
weather softened into Labor Day. Among the diners were a few
businesspeople, but mostly the tables had strollers parked near
them, toddlers playing with spaghetti that cost more than my
month's coffee allowance, or chairs piled with bags—Ann Tay-
lor, Citarella, D'Agostino, Barneys, Duane Reade. There was
the occasional solo, usually smoking and sipping espresso as he
read the *Times* or a thick novel. They looked settled in for the
afternoon. Male or female, they always seemed to be wearing
shorts, loafers, and no socks. Only Europeans took that kind of
time over a meal, even alone in a city of fast turnover. I liked
their leisure and put it aside as a human behavior to study up
on. Take your time. Enjoy, savor, be someone who likes her own
company.

Outside the Atlantic Grill, shaded by forest green umbrellas,
the crowd was more Madison Avenue than Third, more shore
than Adirondacks. An air of reunion hovered over the tables like
the smoke of beach fires, people greeting each other from separate tables. At a corner table near the canvas barricade a very
beautiful woman, maybe sixty, maybe seventy, made me catch
my breath. I stepped out of the flow of pedestrians to inspect
shoes in a window for a closer covert study. She wore her flaw-
lessly white hair in a soft mound, like whipped cream before it's
beaten stiff. Her face was unlined except for faint crow's feet,
and her eyes, when she looked up from her book (a Teddy

Roosevelt biography, I noted with pleasure), had the capacity to flash melancholy or gay in the twitch of a mood. Thin, wearing a white sleeveless shift with a navy blue sweater draped over her shoulders, a double strand of pearls, dark glasses pushed up on her forehead—the clothes were Smith College, Class of '55, but her hair, her kind, youthful face? She was more Lothlórien or Shangri-la than Elizabeth Arden.

A young woman dashed up to the canvas barricade that separated the street from the tables, leaned over, and kissed my fairy queen, taking her by surprise. The interloper (I didn't want to share) was crisp as a celery stalk in navy blue linen shorts and a cream sweater set, a black, sleek pageboy, and pristine espadrilles. Flat espadrilles. The kind they wear in Nice. The kind she probably bought in Nice.

My fairy queen was collected and serene, the interloper was a flurry. I couldn't hear them, but she was yammering as she pulled back from the kiss, flinging her Donna Karan and Stuart Weitzman bags over the barrier into the empty chair, turning to enter the green canvas compound while talking over her shoulder. She sat down and gulped her ice water, her hand furiously flagging a waiter.

Bennington, maybe. Or Goucher. Even Georgetown, if she were a communications major, whatever that is.

I stepped away from the window, the kids' summer shoe sale memorized. My fairy queen reached over to the girl, whose remarks were ping-ponging between the waiter and her companion, and placed her hand on her arm, patted it, and sat back in her chair. The air settled, a drop in decibels. Had a red light halted traffic or a gregarious party left the restuarant? I didn't know, but it was quieter and the umbrellas swelled with sun and glowed. The girl sat back too and folded her hands in her lap as the fairy queen tilted her head and a smile slowly built from her crow's feet to her mouth. She said nothing but the girl's head tilted and I passed them sitting like that, silent, with small smiles of fondness. The interloper had a face full of freckles. She was adorable.

That's *what I want*, I said to myself as the street took up its roar again. *I want a beautiful, calm, content someone to show me how to be the same. I want my clothes and house and friends to be the same when I'm seventy as they are now because they were* always *exactly right.* I might have lost the first forty years of my chance to be a Girl, but when I became one, I wanted to know what was exactly right for exactly me.

I was passing for human, if no one peeled away too many layers. Daily, I was reminded of the baby bird that fell out of its nest in a favorite childhood story, *Are You My Mother?* I was looking for someone to tell me how to live and I would have taken advice from a trombone if I understood what it was saying. Catherine was a Girl I admired and had the workweek's access to. Ten years younger than I, she was a marathon runner, had a slew of best girlfriends, and was in an intense relationship with a man from another city. She'd seen me lose 170 pounds and had heard my quailing uncertainties and realizations and small achievements. For a civilian, she knew me well and I looked to her for advice and close observations, and as a model of how to act on a day-to-day basis.

On the first Saturday night that had something of an autumnal chill, Dennis and I met Catherine and her boyfriend, Stephen, for dinner in Chelsea. It's almost a double date, I told myself excitedly as I got dressed. Three of us are straight, that's almost a double date. I'd never been on a double date. It was so . . . *human*.

Conversation was lively. Dennis had always liked Catherine, and Stephen was cute and smart and obviously prized every twist and trait in Catherine, enough to spend a precious Saturday night with this middle-aged couple who weren't even a couple. Stephen had the aplomb to not make us feel like their parents or faux-hip professors.

By the time our entrees arrived, Dennis had pried out Catherine's childhood on the Main Line, offering her the chance to star in her own *Philadelphia Story*, complete with Peter Duchin and debutante parties. Talking about her Social Register beginnings usually made Catherine squirm, but Dennis was a talented director that night, teasing and milking each tidbit into another admission.

Some of this was familiar turf—Catherine and I were both doctor's daughters. But there were no debutante balls in Missoula, Montana, and private school meant parochial rather than prep academies. I sat back and took notes. Of Catherine's head toss in the story of getting drunk at her mother's Christmas Medical Auxiliary bash in the Temple of Dendur room. Catherine's hair reached the small of her back and had terrific flippability. I flapped my pageboy when she threatened to kill me if I told the story at the office, but it had nothing of the waterfall effect she could produce. I noted how she waved her fork as she talked, ignoring her food. I set my own fork down and made myself take two sips of water between bites. I could at least pretend to be more interested in my companions than in my dinner.

I watched Catherine include Stephen by leaning into him while keeping her eyes on Dennis, and I listened to Stephen laugh as Catherine described a night her mother got so angry at her prep school trash-talk that she locked her out of the house and Catherine climbed back in through a third-story window. *Third story?* I thought. *Where the maid slept?*

"Like mother, like daughter, right, Speedy?" Stephen asked with a grin.

Catherine sat back in her chair, away from Stephen, her arm following the curve of its back. She looked him up and down, as though he were a complete stranger—albeit a Stranger on a Train, a man she could leave everything for after their first meeting.

"Tell Dennis about last Saturday," Stephen went on.

She stuck her tongue out at him and nudged him with her foot. "Fuck you," she laughed. "It's not my fault you finish too fast." She narrowed her eyes in satisfaction at her parry.

Stephen looked at Dennis. "I ran my ten miles and Catherine still had one or two to go. It was hot. I was sweating. But she kept going on the track while I stood there and waited. She had the keys to the house and she'd call out when she passed me, 'I can't stop to give you the keys.' "

"Stopping would have broken my rhythm," Catherine objected.

"As if calling out 'I can't stop, I can't stop' didn't?" Stephen said. Her forearm brushed his, a meaningless collision except that Dennis and I in our years of friendship had no such casual touching. The table vibrated a little. She had scooted her foot over to his.

Their jokes made each other's best stuff better, I noted. Did Dennis and I increase each other like that? We riffed on each other, making tall tales taller, and we discussed. But we did not host one another's absurdities and predilections as delicacies. I flipped my hair and touched Dennis's arm, asking him to tell them about his college "girlfriend" from Nob Hill, his early stab at social climbing and heterosexuality.

It was almost a real date.

The conversation, when Dennis and I came back from a smoke, turned general. I drank coffee as they finished their wine, itchily sorry after watching the pretty people on Eighth Avenue that I'd worn a short dress and tights. Catherine wore black jeans and a plain white T-shirt. She fit in. I felt overdressed but I'd wanted to show off my Girl knees and be a player in the game of going out to dinner on Saturday night. I'd gotten it a little wrong. I made another note to wear black jeans next time.

"I *must* go dancing!" Catherine announced. She reached over for Stephen's quarter-full wineglass. "Where can we go dancing?"

All eyes turned to Dennis.

"What?" he asked. "You think the homosexual knows?"

"It's what we pay you for, dear," I said as I reached over for his half-full ice water.

"I know a club," he relented. "It's a drag show. If it's disco night, there'll be dancing."

It was tiny, tucked into a MacDougal Street wall, raucous with Donna Summer, gay men sizing each other up, and single women with blond teased hair. "Eee-ewe," Dennis scorned. "Jersey girls." A fate worse than death. Now I was glad for my dress and Doc Martens.

Catherine drained a long sip of beer and gave herself up to Thelma Houston, gyrating slinkily amid the flock of luster-headed Jersey girls in studded jeans. She looked good, a free spirit, belonging to no one. Stephen watched with amusement as Dennis yelled in his ear. I nodded my head in time, half rocking my upper torso. I like nothing more than dancing and I wasn't quite sure why I didn't go out there. Partly, it would have felt like competition, trying to keep up with Catherine. It would have felt needy because I'd prefer to dance *with* her and she was obviously alone in the music. And I was sober, with nothing to prove except for everything. The last time I'd been out dancing I'd weighed three-hundred-some pounds, had been drunk, and had a roomful of gay boys join me in the weird ritual rondo of fags and hags. I had been thrilled with my sip of popularity, while the fags were thrilled to be queer but, by association and comparison to me, not freaks.

That wasn't who I was anymore. I wasn't Catherine, either. Tonight I settled for being a spy in the house of Girls. I sipped my club soda and bobbed my shoulders along to "I'm Every Woman." When Dennis went back up to the bar I waggled my glass of ice between two fingers, as Catherine had done with her empty wineglass at the restaurant. *A gesture of command,* I thought, *of desire and thirst and the confidence it would be met.* Something you did with a butler or a boyfriend.

The music segued into the Bee Gees as Catherine continued her circuit of the floor, her arms twisting sinuously as she shook her booty. Once in a while she opened her eyes and smiled at us, at Stephen, before falling back into the song, lip-synching the threadbare lyrics.

What would it take to be in my own skin that thoroughly? Like Catherine, I'd made my rounds of dance floors under dancing lights and emphatically predictable rhythms. That was in my fat days when observers, I would tell myself as I gulped another vodka for Russian courage, could not possibly tell the Girl from the girth. If they had—I squeezed my eyes at the memory—they would have seen a three-hundred-pound ache to be dancing with or for someone. Like Catherine. Like myself tonight, in a body that was no longer a sacrifice to the god of fag hags. Was I ready to live a little dangerously too?

Silence pulsed against us when the music ended and a blue spotlight lit up a red velvet curtain at the back. Catherine kept spinning and spinning, the only dancer. Some of the boys looked at her critically as she threaded through the applause for the patter of a drag queen winding up for her opening number. The singer flung her nylon tresses back with a scarlet dagger of a fingernail, glaring at Catherine in her Bee Gees trance. The karaoke machine played the intro to "Sisters," the boys in their leather and tightly crafted jeans cheered and raised cigarette lighters, and Catherine changed the rhythm of her hips to suit Irving Berlin.

There is nothing sadder, I thought, *than trying to find a beat in Irving Berlin.*

There was nothing sadder than being sober in a club full of bridge and tunnel girls and nostalgic gay men and two fake women who appeared to actually be comfortable in size-14 fire engine red satin come-fuck-me pumps. I gave in to an MGM lion's yawn that was more a gulp for oxygen than the late hour.

There was nothing sadder than morphing into a blob of fat ineptitude because a six-feet-five-inches black man had more hair to flip than I did, and the saucy, sexy skill to make it a statement.

When the Seventh Avenue train decided not to run to Brooklyn, I wandered around looking for a cab in the cavernous streets around City Hall. I thought about Catherine and her groove thang on the dance floor. It was a prodigious performance. She had amused us at dinner with stories of cut-off jeans under her cream-horn debutante gown, then gone on to take the club by its ears and show the frowsy, overripe tunnel girls what dancing really was while braving the fury of a cat-clawed drag queen who did not intend to be upstaged. For an encore she'd thrown up with no apology and none expected. If all that was part of being thin, I was in trouble.

This was more than hair flipping and jiggling an empty glass at one's swain.

This was a rock-hard certainty of who she was, of her right to the music and the response of her body, of her right to be appreciated by all watchers. She had gotten it, I suspected, not from being thin but from having been thin most of her life. I could imitate it, maybe, but I would never assume it as a right.

The drag diva, on the other hand, had turned femininity into a science. Her alien habitation of girlhood was vastly exaggerated, but I could tell that she put on her sequined gown and iron maiden shoes with worship and with the demand that she be worshiped. I could imitate her but I'd be laughed out of countenance for trying.

Nearly psychotic at the hour from my litany of weaknesses, I wanted only to be home for a long, long time. I needed to dance, unseen, to "I Don't Know What to Do Without You." Dance for myself, since there was no one else, dance like it mattered, in the safety of my apartment. At home I could claim my skin, try it out, crazy costume that it was, octopus-confusing with arms and legs and snaps and bra cups that would, when I got it untangled and on straight, make me feel and look fabulous.

"Home," I mouthed silently when the cab dropped me off on Clark Street. "Home." It was Judy Garland's voice, mournful and relieved, waking up a child after being a heroine. "Toto, we're home."

All over the city other women were doing this, too. Trudging home on a deserted street to figure out the girl they wanted to be. The one I chose put on cotton pajamas and flossed her teeth, cued up Urbanized softly enough not to wake the neighbors, swaying to someone else's loneliness with her arms wrapped fiercely around herself. Fierce and tight enough to keep all the fragments together for one more night.

Tired as I was, I was up by six next morning. In losing weight, most mornings I boinged out of bed at four and brewed a pot of coffee while I read for work. By the time I got through my commute I had to pee, as my old friend Tom used to say, so bad I could taste it. That fall it took a vicious turn. With the loss of massive thighs, I couldn't hold it. Several mornings a week I cursed and fumbled at the office door, barging in to fling my briefcase to a reception chair, already reaching for waistbands as I Groucho-walked to the lavatory, emerging with my head hung in chagrin as I retrieved my belongings.

Several mornings a week I wet my pants.

The first time it happened I wailed to Catherine that I had a business lunch.

"Go to Rite Aid."

"I don't want panty liners," I protested. "I have a lunch in midtown. I'll smell like a bag lady."

"Just buy new underwear."

I regarded her blankly. They sell underwear at Rite Aid? How . . . convenient. It hit again, how very easy thin people have it. I'd ordered mine in twelve-packs from Lane Bryant ever since I'd been responsible for my own underwear.

It took a few months to adjust to the mechanics of continence but it is now safe to invite me to sit on your sofa.

Despite my energy, I felt safe only at home, an apartment so small and so lacking in direct light that I couldn't tell the difference between navy blue tights and black. I called it the Bat Cave. In the Bat Cave, my poverty didn't matter, no one was looking at my ill-fitting clothes, I could forget my body altogether in the work—chopping vegetables or reading a manuscript—at hand.

The Bat Cave was a problem in itself, however, a barely functioning refuge decorated in midlife Dorian Gray.

The Bat Cave accrued. Dirt and mildew I hadn't had the mobility to clean, mystery piles that got moved but not untangled. The Bat Cave was the noncorporeal manifestation of my obesity, the same way Dorian Gray's portrait showed the haggardness of his dissipation. Like Dorian, my piles and messes were secret.

Every Stepford has had at least one of these portraits in her home. The first one I tackled, early in abstinence, was by my bed. Books, magazines, notebooks, underwear, sweaters, catalogues, pens, lotion, Cortaid, Post-its, remote controls, VCR and telephone instructions, letters, Kleenex, bookmarks—all the necessities I'd wanted at hand when I spent as much time in bed as possible. As I toiled through the layers I found toenail clippings amid dust bunnies the size of Rome apples among the *Gourmet* subscription inserts. "That was information I didn't need to hear," Katie said with the distaste of someone who cleans behind her refrigerator each week. I was as proud of clearing that pile as I was of losing my first ten pounds.

I had tolerated my moldering portrait because I hid it when company came. No one saw my victory in the first ten pounds or the first sorting and disposing. But I knew. I had claimed a few cubic feet of order on the Planet of Girls.

I wanted to deracinate from the Planet of Fat but every night I came home in my girl clothes to the remains of my origins, on day-release from the Planet of Fat. The Bat Cave, I had to admit, was an addict's dwelling, a crib for overeating. The crumminess had been tolerable because of Entenmann's and because no one really saw or assumed I was capable of anything else. Until I'd hit 168 pounds, I wasn't sure I was, either.

My furniture consisted of crammed bookshelves, a desk, a few uncomfortable straight-backed chairs, a fifteen-year-old futon on the floor with a low easy chair, food-stained and leaking stuffing, at a right angle to it, facing the television. How many nights, just three years ago, had that chair been ground zero? I'd put the exact money by the door buzzer so I wouldn't have to fuss with the deliveryman, waiting in my pajamas so I wouldn't have to disturb myself later for anything as disruptive as getting ready for bed, then leave the dishes and cartons on the floor as I toppled four inches into bed, the remote control set to the Home Shopping Network so I could sneer at call-in customers who peopled their lives with teddy bears by Annette and dolls by Marie.

I wanted to be a writer but I didn't own a typewriter.

Part of being a Girl means living, when no one is watching, like a Girl.

The Bat Cave carries all kinds of metaphorical weight. A crumbling, narrow, groutless box of questionable electrical safety, in the middle of one of New York's prettiest and most expensive neighborhoods, open to a garden that belongs to my neighbors. The Bat Cave personifies the imposture I felt I was, claiming a Brooklyn Heights zip code as I eavesdropped on native Earthlings.

I couldn't afford to move, and I didn't want to. There are things in the Bat Cave's defense. It is on a tree-canopied street. I can hear tugboats and ferries on the East River, the swing sets at the Promenade playground, mourning doves. My dry cleaners know me by name and the men at the newsstand reach for Camel Lights as soon as they see me coming. There is a washer and dryer in the basement. It was my address, a concrete identity for an alien who looks to her possessions—her books, music, tchotchkes—to remind her of who she is.

I didn't have room or money for mission furniture, and I needed a computer. The imperatives were clear: find money, find furniture that fit the space and my needs.

Lists were called for, which always makes me happy. Buy a tape measure; scout futon stores; call Nora about computers; clean; withdraw funds from my retirement account; make sure Nora would help set up the computer and that the two futon frames and computer desk would be assembled. If I had to assemble anything more complicated than a lamp, I'd either have a nervous breakdown or a heap of kindling.

I moved bookcases and thousands of pounds of books, got up close and personal with spots in my apartment I hadn't seen since the first Bush administration. And I could *do* it: bend, hoist, push, climb, lift, kneel, balance, twist. When I finished a task, I'd run out for the little things that would make my habitat more habitable. A mattress pad—why had I allowed my old futon cover to accumulate stains better left unmentioned? Because Macy's, twelve blocks away, was too much of a physical challenge on the Planet of Fat. On the Planet of Girls it was an easy walk in which I was bound to run into friends, or make them. I forged alliances among the small businesses of Brooklyn Heights. John at the mom-and-pop hardware store made me swoon for Rubbermaid, door hooks, stacking hangers, and plastic tubs that fit under my futon couches. He became my surrogate husband, patiently explaining—twice—how to change the cracked toilet seat I'd put up with for a couple of years. Mumbling his instructions over to myself, sure I'd have a geyser in my bathroom, I went home, changed it, and scrubbed the bathroom floor to boot.

My apartment was the first physical challenge of endurance, strength, and flexibility I'd taken on. CD racks and shoe trees got me as high as ketamine.

As a project, it had the beautiful merit of being finishable when so many of the other Girl projects I had to confront were not. I felt purposeful and capable. I envisioned sitting on the couch and reading a book the way I did in my parents' homes, of knowing where the book belonged when I was done.

From addict's crib/Dorian Gray, I passed to living among the blond woods of a college dorm.

It wasn't Stickley, but it was a hell of an improvement.

A woman who is losing weight, or who has become notorious for having done so, puts other women on the defensive. When it comes to a newly thin woman's long relationship with an obese employer, things can get snarky real fast.

Barbara defined me by my size. She may always have defined me by my size—I wouldn't have blamed her. But now I was thin, and she seemed to feel that should have been enough.

One afternoon I went to her to discuss a sticky situation in which I was trying to placate a justifiably upset publisher while negotiating another deal a client had duplicitously sought for the same book.

"I feel dirty from this," I said in disgust.

"You may feel awful, Frahncees, but you look *fabulous*."

The moral of that tale would be that feelings and reputation don't matter when you look good.

Sometimes my weight loss could be part of Barbara's personal bragging rights. One November afternoon, Our Most Famous Client came to visit. I stalled on going up to do the obligatory flattery and was surprised to hear Barbara lumbering down the hall into my office, Famous Client glomping behind her. They piled up in front of my desk. Barbara beamed, turned to Famous Client, and said, without greeting me, "See?"

As I sat feeling like a platypus or a moon rock, Famous Client discoursed on how I would never maintain it, she had never maintained it, and had done the research to know I'd screwed up my metabolism forever. Barbara was no more pleased at the lecture, I think, than I. She'd wanted to demonstrate something—that she had a dynamo on her hands, perhaps, or maybe that hope, for them too, was still alive.

But when I or someone else brought up this thing I had done around Barbara, all hell could break loose. As it did a few weeks later.

I was excited at the prospect of Fredi's visit. Fredi was a well-known editor, enthusiastic and curious. She had always encouraged assistants, her own and me. Now she was the articles editor for a magazine and wanted to discuss our client list. I handled magazine sales and my attendance was required.

Barbara and Fredi had known each other for donkey's years, so I gave them time to chat before joining them, client profiles and legal pad in hand. I was wearing a dress that topped out just above my knees. With my pageboy hair in its usual state of misbehavior, black tights and Doc Martens, I was in full Janeane Garofalo mode.

"Oh. My. God."

Fredi sparkled when she hit on something she could compliment or use.

"Oh. My. God. Look at you! *Look* at you. Frances! You're half your size. Frances, you lost half of yourself."

I smiled nervously and glanced at Barbara, who had pulled back her chair like she had hooked a great white shark in a trout stream. "Not quite." I was scrupulous about the numbers although I knew it would only increase Barbara's ire. "One pound under."

"You're going to write about this, aren't you? You're going to write for *me*!"

Barbara was fuming. My armpits went sour as I calculated what my furniture had cost and how much a winter coat was going to run me, my eyes darting at Barbara. Her mouth had imploded into a rictus that bespoke everything that had hung between us in the last few months. *Isn't it enough that you're thin—what more do you want?* I had done what Barbara wanted to do for herself, but she wanted to be the master of when it could be mentioned. Yet I desperately needed the money, needed the assignment, needed the writing. What could I write for Fredi?

I fluffed the air with one hand, gave a version of "we'll see," and turned the meeting to clients. It went well enough and ended with Barbara and Fredi catching up on their new grandchildren as I fetched Fredi's coat.

Maybe it was twenty feet to the threshold of my office. I got as far as ten.

"Frahncees!" Barbara stopped me. "We really *do* need to talk about your performance with magazine sales."

I pivoted in slow motion.

"There's money to be made here and you simply aren't making it."

I searched her face for how furious she was, how far she might take this. The way her eyes could not meet mine tipped me off.

I considered my responses. I could answer each of these

points. I had answered them in the past. But I was weary of explaining demographics and mandates and time lines and Condé Nast's lack of telephone switchboard operators. And running lightly through my spinning mind was a molecule of insight. I was afraid of Barbara. She could fire me any time she wanted. But she could only do it once, and it would only take a few seconds to do it.

I decided not to cry.

I decided to ask questions.

"Do you feel you and our clients are not informed about submissions?"

"No, that's not it," she answered, her face rumpling to locate the "it" she wanted to hitch me to.

"Am I not making *enough* submissions? Have I advised clients incorrectly on what a magazine proposal is?"

"No, that's not it."

"Do you want me to send stories to magazines that don't publish fiction?"

"You don't know my list," she responded, illogically but with some triumph. "How can you sell my clients when you don't know my list? I know yours."

"Have you given me information about your clients?" I asked carefully. I was treading the line of accusation.

"You should know my list as well as I do yours."

"Yes, I should," I agreed, and paused for her to speak if she wanted. "But then, I give you updated lists of my clients' projects, what's ready to sell, what they're working on next. Do you feel uninformed about them?"

"No, of course not. But it's clear to me that you're only out for your own interests."

Ah. She was teetering toward the crux of it.

"Did I neglect your clients in the meeting with Fredi? What did we talk about for an hour?"

I had created a very dangerous silence. I had a list of Barbara's clients, as well as my own, from whom Fredi was interested in seeing proposals. The truth was worse. We hadn't talked about my clients' interests, we'd talked about *me*.

Fifteen minutes before I should have, I put on my coat and left. On my way out, I saw Barbara hunched over her desk eating crackers like they were coming off an assembly line.

It wasn't a dressing down for bad behavior or lack of effort, I understood by the time I got home and flomped down on my purple futon couch with no intention of picking up a manuscript that night. Barbara had had a tantrum over categories, what I had that she didn't, the haves and the have-nots. Fredi was thin, coiffed, at home in Chanel, and I flat-out adored her. That savoir faire was what I came to the Planet of Girls to find, even if my version was a J. Jill velour dress and dorm room furniture.

I'd been adopted, and by a doyenne at that, into the category of haves, and I'd been asked to document it. Status was at stake where I had been an inferior. Barbara could claim many kudos in the publishing world, but I'd done the one thing she couldn't. I'd lost weight. Driving it home, I had been claimed by an arbiter she, too, admired. And our arbiter had proclaimed me both thin and a writer.

I wanted out. I wanted—everything.

Fredi was my wake-up call.

8

THIS

BODY

It was a wet Friday night in November, the kind of cold that settles in like rust or mildew. Still, it was Friday and around Houston Street everyone was determined to claim it. I was, too. Dennis was back from Italy and we had weeks of travel and news to catch up on.

I was wearing a midnight blue velour jumper I'd bought the winter before. It was too big but the color was rich, engorged, with satin trim at the neck and arms. I liked the sensation of the hem brushing at my ankles and I felt like I was floating into the evening, which was just right for a SoHo reunion. Dennis wanted a drink and we found a bar that we liked the looks of, nondescript and quiet.

It had booths. I adored booths, a cheap trophy of the thin. I fit. Not only that, I could lounge, intimately. My breasts didn't push at the table, I didn't have to inch in and sit at odd angles. I could—this was cool—*lean across the chasm between the seat and table and cross my legs.*

The night was simple. My best friend was home, we had a booth. We had things to say.

But we were hungry and we'd ducked our heads into a restaurant that was dim and interesting and needed investigation. After Dennis's cocktail, we left the bar, linked arms, and headed back to the rosy kookiness of Marion's, only to find every table was taken and the line was three or four groups deep. Dennis spoke to the hostess—Marion herself, as it turned out, the person responsible for the hilarious shrines along the walls. Lassie and Timmy plates and lunch boxes and posters, Jack and Jackie, Scottish terriers. Someone demented created this; we had just met her and we wanted to eat her lamb shanks.

Dennis leaned down. "She can seat us in a minute."

We followed her past the line in front of us, weaving between diners, up rickety stairs to a small table against a railing. It was the bull's eye of the house. I pulled my chair back cautiously, wary in crowded places with wooden chairs and tippy tables that, if I moved them to make room for my belly, could spill water and dump the salt. In this spot, such a mishap could mean calling an ambulance. Another Earth moment: there was room to spare between me and the party behind me.

Dennis leaned over as he unearthed himself from his leather trench coat. "So that was swell, wasn't it?"

"What?" Had he tipped Marion, or said something so infernally wicked that she rewarded us with a table when others were waiting? Dennis had his charms.

"What she said."

"I didn't hear." I was busy arranging my book bag and muffler out of the waiters' paths.

"She said, 'I save this table for pretty people. It draws in the trade.' "

I looked up and smiled. "You *are* pretty. I always say you look wonderfully Edwardian."

"*Frances*. She meant *us*."

Oh.

Was I really one of the "pretty people"? Did this body deserve the privileges eye candy is granted?

"This body" is a phrase I use a lot.

"This body has a big stomach and no hips," I complained to Katie in a morning phone call. I had the same menu to give her as yesterday and my day's food would rattle off faster than a Hail Mary. The morning phone call gave us five or ten minutes to talk about things my precisely formatted food plan kicked up for me. Today I was in a high fine tig over what to wear to work. "Pants fit funny."

Katie objected to my habit of referring to myself in the third person. "Say 'my body.' It's not *this*, it's *yours*."

But saying it—*my body*—was one of the scariest things I had to do. The phrase was too *whole*. With wonder and puzzlement, I was beginning to claim parts of this body with relative equanimity—"my thighs don't meet when I sit," "my feet are so intricate; I never knew they had so many bits and bones." But collecting the parts in "my body" was a claim on something bigger than *me*. I could say "my life" without a blush or a falter; my body was stranger, scarier, than my life. It was as though people would call me on the truth—that I had stashed the other body, my real one, in the back of my closet.

The Stepfords tended to couple the adjective "my" with body types. Katie noted she had a pear-shaped body, while mine, she informed me, was apple-shaped. Bridget, a string bean if ever I saw one, said fiercely, "I have a runner's body." Nora spent months shifting a full-length mirror around her apartment. "I needed to see my body doing various things: sitting and read-ing, washing dishes, whatever," she told me. "I have a dancer's body," Amy justified as she debated the advisability of losing a few pounds her sponsor counseled against.

It was as though someone had gone shopping and picked out these bodies for us, well-intentioned and sometimes brilliantly, but a gift we weren't certain what to do with.

Bridget had her runner's body and Amy her dancer's body; I had a body—and a passion I've been parsing ever since—for clothes.

Consider the old saw "Clothes make the man"—or in this case, woman. Newly arrived on the Planet of Girls, my alien status haunting me, I was a woman very much in need of mak-ing.

"Dear heart," Bridget said as we walked through the last of the leaves in the honeyed thin light of late fall, "you're never go-ing to get real with life if you don't get real with your clothes." She was beautiful when she smiled, as she did then, her auster-ity lifting like the fog had earlier in the day, in a quick steady wisp. This was one of her gentle lectures. She only used "dear heart" when her own was tender, and then there was that smile and crink at the corners of her eyes.

I was dressed for the Saturday morning meeting, wearing my khakis and a sweater my mother had knitted for me years ago, trapezoids of tweedy maroons and teal. It was beautiful. It also drooped to my third knuckles and could house two of me. I was so cold I was glad I could curl my hands up into the sleeves' rel-ative warmth.

"I've got a couple of business outfits," I objected. "I just haven't gotten around to—what do you call clothes you wear on weekends and when you don't have to dress up for work?" Unbidden memories of Ship 'n Shore prizes on late-morning game shows came back to me. Stripy clothes, mix-n-match, five garments that made thirty-six ensembles. "You know what I mean—nice but, like, washable and what you'd wear to the movies?"

"They're called casual clothes, Frances."

"Right. I haven't gotten around to them yet."

"Why not?"

I shoved the right sleeve of my sweater up. It slipped again, Dopey's dangle over the back of my hand. Really, I could keep a Pekingese in that sleeve. Didn't Chinese royalty do that?

"I dunno," I answered, pulling myself away from the thought of a dog's body heat to warm me. "Casual clothes." I shrugged. "That means trousers. Trousers scare me."

Bridget nodded sympathetically. "Of course they do. Go to Eddie Bauer."

"Eddie Bauer makes women's clothes?" I asked. My father used to order hunting clothes from Eddie Bauer.

"Yes, they do. They're classic and they seem to fit our bodies well. Maybe it's middle age, maybe it's the kinds of problem spots we have after losing weight, I don't know. And"—she gave me a salesman's cinch-the-deal grin—"they're *warm*."

As I walked home, I scouted what the women of Brooklyn Heights were wearing that chilly afternoon as they pushed their strollers or swung out of the brunch places with their pals or boyfriends, Gap and Banana Republic bags swooshing. Late November was not a good time for sartorial spying. Everyone was coated and bundled. What I could spy was nondescript. The crisp jeans of women who don't wear them often, leggings and bunchy socks over boots. And no khaki. The season had passed.

But *Eddie Bauer*? I lost 170 pounds for Eddie Bauer? I endured twenty-one months' hunger for rag wool?

Katie always said, "If you want to know why you're eating, stop eating." I'd add, "If you want to know why you're dieting, finish the diet." Bridget was telling me to deal with more of my offstage life—what I looked like on a Saturday.

Every time I leave the Bat Cave, I told myself, *or cross my legs or wrap a bath towel around myself, I'm braving a gauntlet.* Buying pants was no different than dashing out for yogurt without wearing a coat to cover myself up, so off I went. The hardest part was bracing myself against the possibility the clerk would approach and ask, "Are you looking for a *gift?*" which is code to the fat for "What are *you* doing *here?*" I'd never gotten over that expectation, but no one offered more than to take my Visa card. Ten minutes later I was headed back to Brooklyn to Windex my seldom-used closet mirror and assess this body in size 10 corduroys.

I had tried them on. I knew they buttoned and zipped shut; I'd bent over to confirm that I could move. No dressing room, however, gave me the time I needed to fit the parts together into one person, like the children's puzzle that assembles a creature with an ostrich's legs, a pig's body, and a monkey's clever face.

I had to ignore some things about myself if I intended to wear my clothes with confidence. I was tragified at the bit of flesh that flapped over the waist. It was skin rather than fat, but what could I do, wear pants so big from the hips down that I could steam a schooner from Barbados to Nassau with the right wind? Wear a sign: "Skin, Not Fat—Donations Accepted"? I fell back on Lisa's tuck-and-poof, pulling a half inch of shirt over the waistband. One of the bonuses of thinitude, she had told me that summer, was that problem areas could be camouflaged.

As I pushed my conviction that I had a pig's torso aside, I took in the trousers: wide wale, front pleats, cuffed legs. How marvelous! Bridget's "casual clothes" could have the same precision as the business suits she wore. The Planet of Fat used frippery to finish these sorts of clothes, favored by Zaftigs and Perfectionists as announcements of their sensuousness or the image they wanted to perpetrate.

The trousers gave me facts to consider further. Between the corduroy and the pleats, I was all lines. Cool, tidy lines. Tall, I muttered out loud. The cuffed legs emphasized my long legs and knobby ankles. The fit of the legs hinted at the muscle tone underneath. The waist cinched my torso, throwing my breasts into a bas-relief that my suits, with their blazers, didn't show.

So *that's* the deal with the hourglass figure, I realized. It's not the little waist, it's the boobs blooming bigly above it.

Move over, Mitzi Gaynor. I began to hum "There Is Nothin' Like a Dame" and shivered with a wave of pure pleasure at the pool of corduroy, deep as fudge. Fat women get stuck in pinwale, the bulk of this near-velvet too emphatic for the bulk of flesh it can't disguise. I'd favored corduroy when I was fat without realizing it was pinwale. The one garment I'd saved as a reminder of the Planet of Fat was a red pinwale dress I'd worn with a black turtleneck and black tights. Or was it a jumper? My hands paused in brushing my grass-lush thighs and ass as I tried to remember. I'd left the Frances of that dress far behind.

Safe in the Bat Cave, thin was simple. I was swanked in buttery, luxurious corduroy, the material a bit cold and shiny inside, bringing the down on my thighs to prickling alertness. I'd made my stake in my possession of the rolling wide wale terrain of myself, as replete as the fabric implied—the cloth of kings.

I dug around for a trouser hanger to put them away. I clipped one end of the waistband in and the other clip snapped at empty air. I still wasn't accustomed to not folding waistbands in at the seam to hang them up, still wasn't used to how small my clothes were. Fat habits abound.

With a laugh and a last fond petting, I put them away, adding new rules to my guidebook. *Never ever again wear jumpers or pinwale corduroy. No studs, fringe, animal prints, jungle flowers, leggings, tunic sweaters. Never learn to tie a scarf into bouffant origami, never wear wooden beads bigger than decent pearls, never wear earrings wider than their length.*

Not unless I hit size 18 again.

Never hit size 18 again.

. . .

The cords and turtlenecks proved themselves to be warm as the weather petered from stimulating to wretched. Warmth is a constant concern for Stepfords. Many of us never adjust to the loss of the insulation of fat. Whereas summer brought a wave of newcomers who were distraught at what had been under their coats all winter, winter belonged to the regulars. Bridget, Katie, Amy, and I shared secrets of warmth like housewives comparing recipes. When I found glove and sock liners, I bought a set for Katie who had reminded me the day before that a shower would restore sensation in my toes after the commute home from work.

"REI," Bridget told me. "It's a sporting goods company. They make long underwear for ice climbers. Get silk not cotton. It lies flatter under your clothes and doesn't wick."

"Lotion," Katie added, thinking of lard-smeared swimmers of the English Channel. Amy piped up from the depths of a coat that looked like a rag mop on amphetamines. "Look at nature. Feathers and fur, I always say."

Bridget nodded emphatically and trumped us all with a recommendation of vitamin B_{12}. I spent ten months of the year swaddled against breezes and shady streets that normal human thermostats find refreshing. For many months of the year, my Life in the Funhouse Mirror included reminding myself that it was not unreasonable to feel fat and stiff when I was wearing long underwear, Lycra leggings, *and* tights under my wool pants.

It was my autumn of research and observation as I studied how, if clothes make the woman, the details help to complete her.

Clothes taught me things about myself. I was searching for

order and precision and completion; I was searching for sensation and romance. I don't find romance in patterns or frills
(Laura Ashley should remain in the Cotswolds) but I found it in
the valves of motion, in pleats and lines and the sway of fabrics.
I wanted my clothes to purr to the touch.

I dress in solid, mostly primary colors, and this is a key to my
personal aspirations as well. *I yam what I yam.* The more I am
a person like that—true lines and true colors, but a surprise in
a gust of wind or a sudden movement—the truer I feel in the
world.

I have one exception, besides a couple of campy Western
items, to my no-pattern rule. I'm delirious for plaid. Both are
nods to my heritage. If I become aphasic when I have to buy a
sweater or shirt to go with a solid color, I'm a one-woman color
wheel when it comes to plaid. Plaids are the secret I carry—I am
still a St. Anthony's schoolgirl.

I love lines and any and all details that finish clothes in ways
that are impossible in fat clothes: lined jackets and trousers,
belt loops and belts, midi-blazers, and sheer blouses. My preferences in labels, which began with Eddie Bauer and which have
evolved into a full-blown fixation on Donna Karan and the
Spring Street/BoHo designs of Shirley Qian, are not a difficult
exegesis. My clothes draw a hard line, in every kind of way, reminding me not to eat those mashed potatoes, that how I present myself is a choice every day, that I must live up to that
choice.

In cuffed, two-pleated, luxuriously piled corduroys and a
cotton turtleneck, I felt outlined, truthful. Closer to how I
wanted to feel about the person underneath.

.   .   .

A few weeks later, it was Christmastime in Sun City, Arizona, and my parents had invited me to visit them in the home where they spent the winters. I sat drinking coffee and eating an orange from the backyard as Mother described her plans for an open house. She and Daddy were eager to introduce me to their two hundred friends in Arizona; they had ordered that good smoked ham and sent out Christmasy invitations and everyone had accepted.

This wasn't about social obligations or introductions, it was about showing me—my weight loss—off.

We would never admit that, I thought as I examined my cuticles.

"Your nails are long," Mom commented.

"Yeah," I agreed. "I stopped biting them. I should do something with them, they're kind of wild."

Mom reached for the phone. "I have a hair appointment today. Salvatore is dying to meet you. He wants to talk Brooklyn. Let me see if one of the girls can fit you in. It'll be my treat."

And so it happened, amid orange peels and newspapers and the smell of coffee and toast, that Mother and I opened yet another Pandora's box.

I'd never had a manicure, never gotten my nails to the point that I could. I hadn't even considered it when I was fat and it was too mysterious to wrap my already-crazed brain around in my thinitude. It was a Girl Thing I vaguely wondered if I . . . deserved. Manicured nails are a statement of so very many self-conceptions. Manicures say *I'm adult.* They are one more body part taken seriously. They say *I'm worth the money, the time, the attention.* They are frivolous—they make scrubbing the bathroom floor or a burned pan an entirely different matter. I don't know exactly what manicured nails mean in Arizona, but in New York they are a part of the uniform of worker bees who can afford them, along with a good bag and leather gloves.

Above all, manicured nails say *I'm feminine*, in all the shades that can be lacquered onto our sex. Pink—knowingly ingénue: Ginger, June. Fire-engine red—*try* me: Bette, Myrna. Cherry—girl next door: Judy, Rosemary. Ecru—*I care/I don't care*: Katherine, Joan.

The choices of statements were too many and too urgent in the pre-Christmas hive of women. This was my mother's world, the one I remember lying on the bed and watching the preparations for as she and Daddy donned formal clothes for an evening of dancing. The smell of acetone and hair spray summoned other olfactory memories. Chanel No. 5 in cold mink, tinged with cigarette smoke. Shoe polish and Old Spice. The smell of being very small and kissed goodbye, left to the care of my brothers.

Mother always painted on fire-engine red for those nights of dancing. Abashed by the array of boldness at my disposal, I settled on a brownish maroon. Somewhere between Judy Garland and Joan Fontaine.

I watched my nails dry to a dull exsanguinated red as Mother moved through the factory of beauty, leaving me to Salvatore's inquisition on the state of Brooklyn since 1960 when he'd moved out west. I explained that the only expertise I claim of my borough is how to get into Manhattan. The chitchat was on the verge of floundering until he hit on a new topic.

"I could give you a wonderful haircut," he said, lifting the heavy pageboy from my shoulders. "Short. Easy to take care of."

Several considerations went through my brain. The disloyalty to Menarie, my stylist in Brooklyn whose cuts were so good that I needed to have my hair colored more often than trimmed. The expense of coloring that could be eliminated if I cut everything off and let the gray show. My distrust of a different stylist. The rightness, somehow, of doing this. I'd had the same pageboy from a size 32 to size 10. I have hair that stylists yearn to work with: coarse, thick. But it works against itself, as well. Whatever they sculpt with the blow-dryer soon turns to a heavy lank pall.

"Could we cut it so the gray would be part of it?"

"It'll be very chic," Salvatore promised, rubbing his hands. "I would love to cut your hair."

"I'll bet," I said dryly as I followed him to a chair. "I have more hair than you've had in your hands all week."

I shut my eyes and let him do what had to be done. When he was finished and held up a mirror for me to admire his work, I couldn't stop looking at the floor.

"I wonder," I calculated, "how much all that *weighed*."

It was deliciously light. Dad complimented me once and forgot it but Mom continued to snap, crackle, and pop at what she took credit for. It was another of the things that confirmed her part in my losing weight, allowing her to feel that my triumph, as she thought it, was partly owing to her. As it was.

I found I liked my nails, although I disliked the muddy color I'd chosen. I hadn't noticed before that nail salons in New York are as ubiquitous as Starbucks and the Gap, or that this manicure business wasn't all that expensive. Since I couldn't yet own up to Menarie that I'd had my hair cut my someone else, I strolled into a different Montague Street salon on the first Sunday of January and asked for an appointment.

So began my tutelage under Ella, a brisk, stocky woman whose mahogany eyes made up for her bossiness. Immediately, she noticed the flesh hanging from my upper arms and asked how much weight I'd lost. She cocked her head and nodded without comment. The next week, she told me I needed to do something about my eyebrows.

"Oh, no," I gasped, looking at her thin, penciled arches. "I like them heavy. I want Brooke Shields's eyebrows."

"You think Brooke Shields doesn't wax?" Ella rolled her eyes and chin with the crow of dismissal. "You think she does not shape them?" she went on, her Russian getting the better of her English. "You need to clean them up, give them shape. And—" she leaned over the table—"we need to do something about your upper lip."

So now I was Alice B. Toklas? But of course the idea, once it was introduced, that I was sprouting even the faintest mustache, was abhorrent. Anything else was optional: weedy eyebrows, fuzzy legs, the "beard" Lisa noticed when I modeled my swimming suit that summer. But no, emphatically, I was *not* Clark Gable!

I let her heat up her pots and found I rather liked the sensation that I was a cake being slathered in icing. But maybe she was right to lower her voice. "It doesn't hurt," I told friends when I couldn't do something because "I'm off to have all the hair ripped off my body," but it was a little weird. I didn't realize how sensitive my skin was until I had my lip waxed and sported a strawberry Kool-Aid mustache for a day, despite the ice cube I held to it. I'd always wondered if it was true that if you snip off one side of a cat's whiskers, it would lose its balance. I felt off-balance for a day or two after having my lip waxed. I kept touching it to see if it was still there, and I sported a rosiness I would have liked in my cheeks.

Of all the secrets Ella and I came to share—bikini waxes, the dye she applies once a month to my eyebrows and eyelashes, the heavy calluses she shaves off of my feet—it was the faint hairs on my upper lip that she lowered her voice for.

We had come to share those secrets, as well as the events of the week, because she waxed my eyebrows to such remarkable effect. It was not something anyone noticed. When she handed me the mirror, I complimented her handiwork but I didn't see the difference. Until the hairs started growing in. Unless I look at photos such as those taken that Christmas, in which my short hair reveals the length of my face but my eyes are shuttered by brows of mourning.

That finishing touch opened up my face, turned my eyes from an indeterminate dark to a visible blue that morphed, I learned as people began to compliment my eyes, gray or navy or violet or green. I chalked up this unsolicited poll to my moods and what I was wearing and went with my driver's license description of dark blue. I did know I looked fierce under my new eyebrows. They popped my face into an intent it didn't have before. Sometimes I thought they made me devilish, and that was OK, too.

It was, once again, the 6:55 A.M. call to Katie. I was triumphant about some new purchase. "The first time I tried on size 10 jeans and they fit," she recalled, "I hyperventilated. I had to leave the dressing room and call my sponsor."

I nearly moaned in relieved recognition but she had more to say. "Have you considered that mirrors and reactions have gotten too important, Frances? You'll figure it out by trial and error, and it'll go faster if you pay attention to something besides what you look like."

I tapped a pen on my desktop. This wasn't just about vanity, it was wondering if I really *was* Ralph Lauren or ought to transform myself according to Fredi's epiphany over lunch: "You look just like Cokie Roberts!"

"What are you suggesting?" I asked. "Do you want me to read to the blind?"

Katie sighed. "Start closer to home. Think about how someone else looks. You have enormous experience to offer someone, especially if they come from big numbers. Put your hand up. Volunteer to sponsor."

That Saturday I looked around the Rooms. There were a number of faces as scared and confused as mine had been. I didn't know if I could handle someone's terror and despair. What, I searched my memory, had drawn me so inexorably to Katie?

I had whispered to her early in our acquaintance that one reason I wanted her was because "I think I might be pretty, too." I'd been as afraid and ashamed of that as I was of my pulchritude. Katie had nodded, knowing that pretty on top of newly thin would be another complication on the Planet of Girls.

Maybe I could help someone face the prettiness she'd swallowed along with all the Sara Lee.

I'm a snob, I realized. *I don't really like fat people much. I want a pretty sponsee, someone I can be proud of.* I shook my head in disgust with myself but there it was. And a prejudice was no excuse for not helping someone. Pretty women needed sponsors as much as drab ones.

I'd looked for someone who had what I wanted and asked her how she was achieving it when I called Katie twenty months earlier. There is no official line on choosing a sponsee but I applied the same principle. The only woman who had what I wanted to encourage was that blonde, the Zaftig who came in late and sat at the bottom of the circle. Pam. She was pretty, sociable, spoke with a tough humor, and was miserable about her big weight. I decided to tell Pam how to lose weight.

I corraled her after the meeting with a compliment. "You are *so* beautiful. I hope you know how beautiful you are?"

She smiled a smile as bright as a fresh bottle of seltzer, pleasure and gratitude snapping in her eyes at the infusion of oxygen. I rarely spoke to people I didn't know, and it was hard to get to know me, even in the Rooms where becoming known was the point. I stuck with my cousins and aunties clustered around Katie and Bridget, women who shared my food plan. But I was also the poster girl of weight loss. Everyone knew that much about me, whether they thought I was an ice princess or not. Being approached by a princess, cold or warm, had its flatteries. This tall woman, well over three hundred pounds, was gratified that I'd left Tracy and Bridget at the church gate to initiate a conversation with her.

I plunged on, not wanting to appear smug. "I notice you raised your hand for a sponsor. Do you want to talk about that sometime?"

"Do you want to have coffee?" she asked.

I blinked. People put their lives in strangers' hands so quickly, so trustingly, in these Rooms. I didn't know whether it was appalling or amazing. I looked down at my Hush Puppy oxfords and the cuffs of my black cords. I said yes.

Pam wanted what I had because she thought I was thin and successful. I let her have her fantasy. She did not, however, want my food plan.

I went to work on the pitch. "Weighing and measuring is the perfect metaphor for living. Weighing and measuring time, grief, fun. We're addicts. We never know when enough is enough."

"I just got off sugar and that was hard. You want me to eat how much salad?"

"You'll get used to it. It's quite portable. I eat out for work all the time and I lost 170 pounds in just over a year."

Her sigh turned wistful at that. "God," she said shakily. "I know my arthritis will be easier if I get the weight off this body. If I just wasn't so big."

"This body" got my attention. "Tell me about that. What do you want out of being thin?"

She thought a moment. "To feel better. I know my allergies and asthma are worse because I'm heavy. I'm worried about job hunting looking like this. What will they think? Do I have the energy to work?" She paused again. "And to wear a white

T-shirt tucked into blue jeans." She looked me dead in the eye. We had all come into this church with a vision of unremark-ableness as our highest goal. I'd had Janeane Garofolo, she had Cheryl Tiegs.

"Then weigh and measure. You'll lose weight fast and you'll feel better almost immediately, I promise."

We began the next day. It was peculiar, being bursar to an alien stepping up to the spaceship. I warned her about the diar-rhea that comes with shifting to pounds of vegetables a day, reminding her that every run to the bathroom would show up on the scale. I suggested whole fruits instead of juice, recom-mended goofy coffees that provided a hint of the desserts she'd left behind, explained how salt drew out the water in her salad, helping to disperse the dressing. Three days into it she'd looked around at her apartment and announced, "I'm a messaholic." Her coffee table, she reported, was heaped with magazines, cat-alogues she couldn't afford to shop from but couldn't let go of the possibilities they contained, nail polish and its kindred sharp instruments, coffee cups and napkins and Kleenex, re-ceipts, bankruptcy paperwork mingling with grocery lists and birthday cards and bills and the *Times* help-wanted section from several Sundays ago, ashtrays, and empty prescription vials.

Welcome to the attic of Dorian Gray.

"Uh-huh." I laughed in recognition. "So clean the coffee table."

"I tried," she said. "But I couldn't see any difference. It's de-pressing."

"Set the timer for fifteen minutes and work until it goes off," I told her. "Do it every day and you'll see progress. It's like los-ing weight."

"Ohhhh," she said in the mocking innocence I was getting to know well. "So that's how it works. A day at a time and I'll be you."

"Oh, God, I hope not." It was bad enough to wake up to this

body and this life of mine once a day. I couldn't see how Katie put up with it and I certainly didn't want it echoed back from Pam. "You'll end up at lower-middle-class wages with a boss who scares you, and a nervous breakdown every time you have to get dressed. For fifteen minutes a day let's talk about your body and forget about my life, OK?"

9

HABITAT

FOR HUMANITY

My motives in going after Pam were screwy and layered in my many vanities, but inasmuch as asking Katie to sponsor me was asking to join *in*, offering to sponsor Pam was inviting a stranger to join *me*. It was part of a continuum.

I listened not only to how she wanted more oil on her salad but to her problems. They gushed out in a stream of anxiety, putting my own problems in the perspective of being luxuries. What to wear, how to deal with Barbara and clients were simple compared to Pam's pending divorce, bankruptcy, lack of health insurance, lawsuit, dwindling unemployment compensation, job search, boyfriends, allergies, infirmities, and her sixty-seven best friends who got to eat whatever they wanted.

With enormous reluctance, I had to admit how lucky I was.

I couldn't fix her life, but I could tell her not to eat over it and to take the lessons of the ounces-and-cup measures we lived by into bankruptcy court. "Do an hour's worth of paperwork," I advised. "Then put it away and do something else."

Pam's weight loss was quickly usurping my poster girl status. At six months, she'd lost seventy pounds. Out of work, at the end of her unemployment, looking for a job, clothes were now Pam's, rather than my, crisis.

They say you can't keep your recovery unless you give it away. The thinking is that if you share your experience and tools for success, you will keep them fresh for your own sake. I'd taken a literal approach to finding a sponsor and a sponsee so it was natural for me to be literal in giving away my recovery. I decided to give Pam my clothes. If the 32s and 20s were gone, I'd be that much more reluctant to gain the weight back.

"I can sit and read in the kitchen while you try things on," I offered as I opened storage boxes and garbage bags. "You can call me in if you want an opinion."

Pam paused in pulling off her jeans. "Why would you stay in the kitchen?"

"For privacy?"

She laughed her big Pam laugh. "Go on," she joshed. "It's no big deal," and she whipped off her T-shirt. "The only big deal is this," she added, looking down at her belly, "and it's a lot less than it used to be. What first?"

I reached into a box and pulled out a hound's-tooth shorts suit. "I loved this," I said. "It wrinkles easily but you can wear it with white hose to work."

"Oooh," she crooned, reaching for it. "A weskit. Very nice." *Weskit?* I thought as I made agreeing noises. *So that's what that vest thing is.*

Pam had lots of Girl Things to teach me.

Lickety-split she had it on and was standing in front of my closet mirror, straining to see herself from all possible angles.

Two boxes and a garbage bag later, Pam needed a break. She sat down in her underwear and lit up a cigarette.

"It's weird to see my clothes on you," I said as I poured us each a cup of coffee. "They really point out the differences in body types."

"I know. I have a huge ass and breasts. Your dresses work but not the pants." She sighed. "What can I say? My body is what it is." She took a deep draw on her cigarette. I admired the lipstick stain it left on the filter, the hollow *pwf* and slow exhalation. It was very feminine, and suddenly, her nearly nude Rubenesque lack of shame in this pause between boxes broke my heart.

"I really appreciate your . . ." I searched for words, watching her reaction carefully, "um, *frankness* about taking off your clothes in front of me."

"Why?" she asked sharply.

"It's hard for me to take my clothes off for anyone. I hate what I did to my body. No matter how good I look dressed, I'm a freak under my clothes. It's instructive to see you so casual about it."

"Oh, honey," she said. "If I let myself worry about all this—" she opened arms to display her girth and its damages to her skin and muscles "—I'd never be intimate. You know. With a man, but with you, too."

I nodded and smiled, sadly or humbly. Pam's fifteen minutes in the morning had brought us to this Lane Bryant moment. Sharing clothes was an act of sisterhood. I'd wanted a sister almost as much as an endless supply of cupcakes when I was a kid—this was an old wish fulfilled. I had ungrown my clothes but Pam was teaching my heart to be large.

We belonged to each other.

· · ·

Remember the calculus-nerd cajoled onto the basketball team because of his height? Never, once, had I been argued into a sport, and I knew that if I was, I'd be as disastrous as he, tipping the ball into the other team's basket and stumbling down the court, shoelaces flapping. And yet here I was: long, tall, strong legs, knee-jiggling energy.

That was when Katie started in, during my morning phone calls.

"I hear an awful lot of rushing around," she said. "When did you get up this morning?"

It was a Saturday. Saner people had given in to the wear and tear of the workweek on Saturday, but not me. I couldn't. "I don't know. Four? I need to get organized. I found *three* watches, perfectly good ones, that need batteries. And terrific shoes that are all frayed and lopsided. They're lovely, Kate. Maroon suede—"

She cut me off. "You're packing your weekends, aren't you?"

"I can only do it then. The hardware store closes at six and I need to put everything away—"

"Running, running. How do you feel on Monday morning after all that?"

The mention of Monday deflated me. "Why ask? You already know. The office. What's Barbara's mood going to be? Will I get in trouble for going downtown to lunch? Will some client call in a huff because I never got a response on a magazine proposal?"

"Mm-hm," she said. "The weekends are all running around and the weeks are all anxiety. What does that tell you?"

I reached for a cigarette, an eye on the clock. It was eight o'clock in the morning, the weather finally warming up as St. Patrick's Day approached. I wanted to get to Macy's early. I wanted new bath mats. "Uh . . . that I want to be a housewife?"

"Maybe. But you're bouncing with energy and worry. There's only one place I've found to balance all that out."

"Meetings?"

"This is raw energy, Frances. You can't put this into words until you do something physical with it. It's time you start thinking about the gym."

The first four notes of Beethoven's Symphony no. 5 tolled with this pronouncement.

For 173 pounds, I'd stonily resisted all the perky questions about exercise, bragging that I did it with food and the subways—my taxi receipts dropped fifteen hundred dollars in the first year of the diet. "You have to exercise," interlocutors informed me. "It'll tighten up your skin." I quoted my father on Popeye. That skin wasn't going anywhere. Sometimes they believed me and sometimes they stuck by their myth of the gym as the cure for all pestilence.

My stubbornness had several sources. My biggest fear was that I would break the equipment. I had a history of being escorted to a special scale that weighed beyond 320 pounds; I'd splintered office chairs into clanging hardware, and had had medical technicians fret that I wouldn't fit their MRI machines. My father had splinted my bed with steel braces. My fear of breakage was well grounded.

Katie had tried this gambit before, but gently, wisely seeing that the diet and weight loss had been enough for me to deal with. Now, however, with physical zoom added to my whirlwind worries of work and chores, she was adamant.

"You'll feel better, Frances. You need to work out some of this frenzy. And there are some things you can tone up."

I had a thesaurus of excuses. I would look foolish. Worse, I would look grotesque. I would heave and pant and *sweat* while everyone else was humming along like spokespeople for Arrid Extra Dry. I—my arms, my thighs, my gut—would jiggle. I had visions of a skinny aerobics teacher in pink Spandex screaming, "Faster, Frances! Pump those legs!" and screaming back, "*Finnegan's Wake*, Tiffany! Raise that IQ!"

I wasn't any better at working gizmos than I was at assembling or fitting them. I might have to ask questions. Hadn't I asked enough by making friends with John at the hardware store? Hadn't I admitted my stupidity in calling the Stepfords about everything from what to eat, to how to handle Barbara, to setting up my computer?

"I wouldn't know what to *do* there," I whined.

"It's like riding a bike, Frances. In fact it *is* riding a bike." She paused to giggle. "You do know how to ride a bike, don't you?"

"Yes," I drawled.

"I know you can swim—how hard is that?"

"Locker room, men at the pool, *finding* the pool," I began enumerating.

Katie laughed at my blunderbuss. "You're a smart girl, Frances. You'll figure it out. Or don't if you don't want to. I just know how I feel when I leave the gym. Calmer. Better. You don't have to do anything hard. Someone will show you how to use the equipment."

If the time was ever going to come that I'd have the gazillion dollars I figured a gym membership would cost, it was that spring when I was still flush with funds I'd withdrawn from my retirement plan.

I took it under advisement.

I added the gym to my list of things to do.

I promptly refined my talents for procrastination. Behind my excuses of an urgent manuscript to read or late nights at the office was the problem of leaving my apartment for new and hyper-physical scenery. I wouldn't pass in the gym. It wouldn't be a matter of how I looked but of what I could do. Was I strong enough? Could I endure? Would I keep challenging myself, further, faster, longer? Would I give up on it, would I be consistent? The gym was harder than starting a diet. I knew how to be hungry and I could be hungry at home. I could be hungry without anyone knowing. Going to the gym would not be secret.

At dawn and after work, people trickled along my street toward the gym. I picked them out easily: springy sneakers and Lycra, high-tops and baggy shorts, whatever. I admired their discipline and envied them the pause they carved out in their days, the serenity implied in their yoga mats and Walkmans. My days were packed with tasks and errands, meant to produce things. The gym, I argued, would be frustratingly ongoing. I would never finish it. I would never get a concrete *thing* from it—except my body. And there was the rub. I would meet my body there. A blind date on a stationary bike.

The gym met my theory of conveniences, which I had allowed to dominate my choices since joining the Stepfords. It goes like this: if a thing I needed to do was within six blocks, I had no excuse for not doing it. The Stepfords met two blocks away; the gym was less than a cigarette away.

I made the call.

"What took you so long?" the staff member who enrolled me asked when I gave him my address. "Shame on you!"

Mission one accomplished. I deserved a break.

I sorted books and CDs, alphabetized my apartment, ironed, minced cabbage—anything sensible that would put off tying on my sneakers and getting them soiled in the one block to Clark Street.

I talked to the Stepfords about it.

Tracy and I confided our naughtiness as Stepfords on a regular basis. It was our misfortune that we came up through parochial schools in the last of the golden age when Haley Mills was every girl's idol. There is an art, endemic to Catholic schools, to being bad and getting away with it, and a code of honor to protect the backs of one's peers who are pulling off their own feats of badosity. As Stepfords, it took the form of confessing that we were deviating from our proscribed habits ("I can't *stand* that damned morning meditation book," I told Tracy on the phone as I was ironing. "When does 'program' turn into 'programming'?") or checking out food choices ("Whaddaya think, Frances? Is margarine on my rice cake OK?").

Sometimes it was shopping. Tracy was my partner in sartorial crime.

She had steered me into an Orchard Street cubbyhole and zeroed in on a wall full of sweaters. I was oblivious, talking about my gym-ambivalence. "It's one more thing, you know? On top of reading for work and going to meetings. I just want to go home at night."

"You'd look great in this." She started shoving my arms into a coral sweater. "I know how you feel. Bridget's trying to get me to go, too. I joined but I've never been."

"You joined a gym?" It was a betrayal.

"A month ago. I can't get myself to go."

It wasn't a matter of laziness, Tracy had more energy than anyone I'd ever met. For other people. She kept her big Italian family as happy as they were capable of being, cosseted her nursing staff with pastries she couldn't eat, and made the wards under her supervision profitable to the hospital CEOs. Her house was surgically clean, every wall hand-stenciled and every chair covered in cabbage roses, the bathrooms fulsome with embroidered "hostess" towels, embossed soaps, and cranberry candles. If Martha Stewart and Laura Ashley got together over some really good hashish, they'd come up with Tracy's house.

Tracy was definitely one of the Perfectionists. Eating was her consolation for how much of herself she gave away. She refueled by eating out of the refrigerator at three in the morning after having rebottled her spices in matching Lillian Vernon jars and ironing the kids' jeans.

"So why don't you go?" I asked.

Her red curls bobbed as she studied the price tag. "This is only twenty dollars, baby. You definitely gotta get it. I'm talking to my therapist about it," she rushed on. "He thinks it's rebellion. I'm so tired, Frances, of always doing things for people." The way she said "tired" squeezed my heart. She really was tired, empty. "Bridget tells me what to eat and everything I gotta do for program and it's like the gym is one more thing I have to do for someone else. I joined because I'm a good girl, but I can't go because I'm a bad girl."

The next week I decided to follow the Nile—or the Nike—to its source. I asked Bridget to lunch.

This was risky. Not only would she scrutinize my food, but if she said I had to go, I'd have to go. As my grandsponsor, Bridget was another boss of me.

Bridget had been emphatically against exercise for more than ten years of her weight loss and maintenance, and in my early days among the Stepfords I had taken comfort in her 160-pound achievement without a single squat-thrust. In the last year, however, she had reneged and turned into the Amelia Earhart of the treadmill.

"It's just me," she cautioned in meetings as she described the joy of running. "It works for me." So despite making Tracy join a gym, she might stick to her "do whatever works for you" policy. Maybe she would inspire me. Or maybe she would command it. Then I'd be back to confessing my naughtiness to Tracy again.

I was relieved when she ordered a chef's salad. I did so as well, looking forward to the ham and cheese, foods I never had at home. I rotated my Diet Coke in its ring of condensation as we handed our menus back to the waiter.

"I was thinking about getting to the gym this week. Check out the facility, see what's what. But it's one more thing to do and I'm working all the time as it is."

Bridget clapped her hands and beamed. "You'll love it. I run every noon at the gym near work. It's the best feeling I've ever had and I wish I'd found it years ago. You have to get a trainer. A trainer will set up a regimen and push you."

Yikes! I winced. Getting a trainer was even more heroic than just going to the gym. A trainer meant asking questions, asking for help, being inspected for every muscle you moved. It meant inviting a stranger to study your body. Another Perfectionist, her glowing enthusiasm caused another clutch of my heart. Bridget lived in knots, over work, over food, over where to vacation, and the precise cross between oyster and off-white she wanted for her living room light switches. Bridget wasn't just serious, she was grim. Laughter and relaxation were learned skills for her. Exuberance—from a treadmill!—was like watching Mr. Spock fall in love.

I grumped on my way home, one eye on the people obviously headed for the gym. What does she know? She could afford a trainer to direct her regime.

I called Nora.

"It's scary," she reassured me. "When I went back to the gym after losing the weight, I cried. Something about formal exercise just opens a hole in my chest. And you know, it's weird because I used to go to three aerobics classes on Saturdays when I weighed 220 pounds, then binge all night. Maybe it reminds me of the binges. But then, what doesn't? I go into the corner bodega or the drugstore all the time, and you *know* what I used to do there. It's not like I'm inactive. I take long walks with the dog and I ride my bike to work, but the gym . . ." Her voice trailed off.

Nora was one of the Drab ones in her eating days, lurking in backgrounds, quiet until an inexplicable explosion of pent-up anger forever docked her as crazy. Her history was a fascinating mixture of asserting her body (who does step class at 220 pounds?) and denial of it. Now very thin, she kept her hair short and her color schemes ran not to a season but to boot camp: olive green, beige, gray. I once sat behind her and noticed her Lane Bryant sweater, a size 16. "You weigh 145 pounds," I informed her. "Get rid of the sweater." Nora could spend weeks debating whether to buy a dress she liked, her brain in smithereens because she'd have to let go of money and she'd look like a Girl, God help her on both counts.

God help me from getting that sphinctered, I thought as I placed the phone back in its cradle.

Tracy had a neurosis going, Bridget an addiction, and Nora a phobia.

I didn't want to develop any of these things, although I understood them all.

Nora called back a few days later to see if I'd sucked it up to walk the one block to the gym. We encouraged and braced each other a lot in the small defeats we perceived in our bodies. Colds, various pangs, tiredness are dangerous territories albeit natural. I call it fat hangover. Anything that catapults us back into a state of mind or body that makes us feel the way we did when we were fat—sweaty, out of breath, judged, slow, cocooned at home, achy—is too real for us: we are beamed back to the Planet of Fat at the speed of light.

"Just go in," she bucked me up. "If all you do is make it past the front door, you can say you've been in the gym."

I could do that.

The following Saturday, an hour before the gym closed, thinking that most people would be home getting ready for their glamorous evenings out, I wrestled myself into my new sports bra. If all I did was find out where the bikes were, I'd have done it. I could say I'd gone to the gym. I'd know where to go next time.

I tossed half my cigarette away, to the grimace of a svelte woman my age coming out of the building, gym bag slung over her shoulder. She was wearing a sports bra and no shirt. Shit. I looked at the cigarette in the gutter, sighed, and turned to the big glass doors. It was an effort to push them open. Maybe I did need the gym.

"Hi," I said to the drowsy college student at the front desk. "I just joined. What do I do now?"

She gazed mutely at me. Maybe I should go home and wait for a graduate student to take over the desk.

"Uh, well, what do want to do?"

The uneven bars? Javelin?

"Uh, well, hmm. Ride a bike?"

"OK. What's your membership number?"

Bad question. I am allergic to numbers. I repeat phone numbers because numbers make my brain cells fly in all directions. I'd lost the rhythm of my chanted membership number they'd given me when I paid my dues with the evil look from Buff Lady outside.

I tried.

"Nope," she said, gazing into her computer screen. "It's not in here. What's your last name?"

Better question. I'd been spelling for quite some time. I was in.

I was in a lobby, with big comfy seats and a juice bar off to one side. Where were the bikes? I took a long look around the parlor. Wheat grass juice but no bikes.

"The women's locker room is right there," the desk girl said. "You can get a towel just inside and use an empty locker."

I gave her the silent gaze she'd given me when my number didn't come up. I'd "done" locker rooms in high school. A shower after PE was mandatory, except when we had our periods or plantars warts. What with one or the other, the gym teachers must have worried that I was anemic and crippled by the time I fell into my junior year.

"I don't need— I'm already— Another time— Wherearethebikesplease?"

"Upstairs." I took a step toward the staircase beyond the locker room. "Or downstairs." We were doing the Scarecrow on the Yellow Brick Road here. I wanted badly to lay down on one of the deep leatherette couches and cry.

Another deep breath, big enough for a quick eenie-meenie. "I see upstairs. Where's down?" She pointed. I went.

Into, it seemed, the bowels of the Wicked Witch of the West's dungeons, where flying monkeys torture little girls and yappy

dogs. Gleaming machines with drawings of the human muscu-
lature in bright red, muscles I doubted I possessed or could pro-
nounce. There was a bike in the big white room of mirrors. It
had a sign. "Five Minutes Only." Wow. One calorie.

As I stood reading the sign and wondering what it would be
like to be crushed by one of these monstrosities, a staff member
happened by.

"Trying to decide what to do first?"

"First and last. I just wanna ride a bike. There's a five-minute
limit, though."

She laughed. "This bike is for cool-downs after weights. There
are bikes downstairs you can ride for as long as you want." I
looked at her more closely. I was home. She was all Irish, from
her red curly hair to her green eyes to her big grin.

"My name is Frances. I just joined."

"I'm Colleen. And don't worry, it's just like every gym you've
been to before."

Now I laughed. "No. I've never been to a gym before. Well,
not since volleyball, and they made me play with special ed
girls."

"Ah. So you want to ride a bike. Let's go."

Colleen trotted me down more stairs, to a running track that
bordered a basketball court. Two sides were lined with bikes,
treadmills, and something I suspected was a StairMaster. I knew
about Stairmasters. I'd seen one on *Sex and the City*.

But the treadmills . . . "How do you do the treadmill?" I
asked, piqued beyond my diffidence. Real Girls, sporty Girls,
talked about treadmills as much as they talked about boys,
calories, and the Gap.

"Can you set them really slow?" I asked.

"As slow as you want," Colleen said, and shepherded me
over. Down the rank of planks an elderly man plodded along,
last week's Sunday *Times Magazine* propped up in front of him.
I turned back to Colleen. She stopped in her instructions about
manual settings.

"You can *read* on a treadmill?" I had a moraine of *New Yorkers* at home. Stacked on the floor, they were land mines. I'd take a step toward my desk in my stocking feet, hit one, and surf all the way to the window. This could be three-for-the-price-of-one. Get fit, get smart, and clean house all at once.

Quite a bargain at that rate.

Colleen bumped the speed up from .2 miles an hour to 4, asking me questions as I found, for the first time in my life, a stride. How could I not have been in a gym before? I gave her a quick tour of my interstellar migration, and at the mention of the Stepfords a beatific peace settled across her pixie's face.

"I see. You know, I have always wanted to be a trainer. I love being fit. It wasn't until I went into recovery that I went to school and got certified."

We held each other's eyes a moment. "Friend of Bill's?" I asked, referring to Bill Wilson, the cofounder of Alcoholics Anonymous and the superego of all twelve-step programs.

"Three years sober. You're going to come back, aren't you?"

"Tomorrow," I promised.

I used Colleen's journey to the gym, part of her recovery of herself, to make myself go back there. The weight room still gave me the heebie-jeebies, but I knew how to work the treadmill and the bikes, and I could prop up a magazine and take in the strange scene in small sips. It made sense that it was reading that allowed me to establish a routine—hadn't I always viewed the world through words?

Lying under *Talk of the Town* was a screen that made interesting designs as I experimented with speeds and inclines, and I liked seeing the graph of what I had done at the end of the half hour we were permitted on the equipment. A new numbers game! How many circuits could I do on the treadmill? How many miles? How many bursts in speed that had me running or what inclines to boost calories burned?

Actually seeing what I could make of my time got me spying on other bodies, other capabilities. I am a horrible snoop, unsure what "normal" is, what is "acceptable." Of course I wanted to be one of those fleet, sleek girls zoned-out on endorphins and the inspiring beat of their Walkmans. I envied their long strides and flipping ponytails. I admired what was obviously an ingrained routine for them, towels draped over the readouts so they could sneak extra time, Poland Spring at the ready. I knew better than to bring refreshments and electronics along: the first time I thought I'd matched my pace to the treadmill's and closed my eyes, I'd gone shooting off like a rejected can of Jolly Green Giant peas. I went back to obsessing about numbers with my eyes open after that.

This was the first time I'd counted calories in the twenty-six months I'd been with the Stepfords; even Katie admitted that, at the gym, calories were Salome's Dance of the Seven Veils.

The other side of my mania was the peace I found on the treadmill. At about eight minutes I began to sweat, the first time I'd ever courted sweat, once I saw that everyone else was sweating too, that sweat was the point. At twenty-two minutes, my mind shifted into a state I'd never experienced, less the endorphin rush I'd heard about than a sense of well-being. I floated when I left the treadmill. A bad day and the treadmill were meant for each other. The treadmill before any day was a good idea. I found a calm there I didn't get from human interaction or a hundred repetitions of the Serenity Prayer—stately, organic, coursing through me like a slow drug.

Who knew that an hour in the gym paid off with two hours' more energy in the evening? Who knew that swinging my arms (something I carefully eschewed because it took up more space on a sidewalk) would help me run?

I loved being able to say, "I've got to go to the gym tonight," joining the haste of my neighborhood in getting home to change out of our business suits and scooting out before supper and *Seinfeld*. It was an incantation of strength and discipline, it said I was in control of my body. "I gotta get to the gym" was millennial code for "I'm pissed off and I'm gonna do something about it." Something, for me, besides eat or brood. "I gotta get to the gym" was saying "I'm going to disappear," into a place no one could follow, different from other disappearances. "I'm going home" had a note of collapse; "I'm going to the movies" invited the argument that I didn't deserve a treat. But the gym claimed health and sanity. No one argued with it. Even bosses respected its invocation.

The world was divided into members and nonmembers, and members had special dispensation. Active but individual; each had her own agenda in the gym. Girlhood is picking and choosing, and I wanted to be one of *those* girls.

Only very occasionally did the gym make me crazier walking out than going in.

I had taken a long hiatus from the gym but had told Nora I was going back. She was, as always, encouraging. "Easy does it," she said that afternoon. "You have nothing to prove. Become a marathoner next week." I took her advice. Walking in would be enough, and that night was about getting my hot horny angry blood flowing, and maybe a little sweat against the early April chill.

I arrived, no *New Yorker* to entertain me, and took a treadmill facing the basketball court. It was less bunny-filled than the room upstairs with its subtitled CNN and patter on the his-and-her bikes. I liked watching the courts, the tussles and politics of basketball. I started out at 3.5 miles per hour, my usual speed, got an incline going, got involved in how well the shrimpy fourteen-year-old was playing against the behemoths. I was out-pacing the machine and I bumped it up, some more, more again, until I was comfortable. I found my natural rhythm at the next level.

I looked up from the readout to see myself in the Plexiglas. What a getup! Knee-length skins, ankle socks, sneakers, a baggy T-shirt. There was nothing pretty there but the thing was, I had *no thighs*. They didn't touch. At all. I was startled because they should have been quaking at that speed. They weren't. They were hard and honed. *I* was hard and honed. I was so mesmer-ized that I didn't notice that the game was over until I felt a shift in atmosphere. Two or three guys were fooling around at the basket at my end of the court, watching. The guys in the work-out room behind me were fooling around, watching.

Me.

Watching me.

It wasn't leering. It wasn't disgust. It wasn't even curiosity. It was a kind of unthinking idle interest: nothing better to do than dribble this ball and watch the treadmills, which were empty except for me. I looked at myself in the Plexiglas again. Big shirt, flat chest, tight slim thighs, long legs, chin-length hair go-ing flat with sweat, long parentheses grooved around her mouth, definitely not young, definitely not a gym bunny. So what was the deal?

I called Nora when I got home.

"I get why the gym terrifies us," I announced. "When you've lived far away from any part of your body besides your mouth, *everything* about your body is a sensation. I can't fucking cross my legs without wanting to call the *Times*. The gym is sensory overload. It's *all* body but it's all *thin* body. We're thin and the gym is the place where that's definitive and revealed. We're not pretending, we're not passing. *We* are thin, not our clothes. We *are* our bodies, in a place where *everyone* is their body. Next to sex"—we giggled a little hysterically at the rumor of the theory of sex—"it's the ultimate reality."

"That's it!" she cried in a kind of relief. "You've *said* it. That's the thing about the gym."

Nora has an active life. She jogs in Prospect Park, rides her bike, doodles around on Roller Blades, but she hasn't gotten over her gym phobia. I couldn't blame her. Taken in too consciously, without the promise of a binge or the focus of a magazine, our bodies and their abilities are on open display.

Katie had one other membership to offer, by precept rather than suggestion. Part of her weekend madness, along with food foraging, the Stepfords, cleaning, and the gym, was church. She and her fiancé were active in their congregation. I'd heard about her choir's *Messiah* at Easter, about the search for a new pastor. I heard and I shrugged it off. Choir was an activity of my childhood, in which I'd sung treacley folk songs in order to get out of math class for funerals.

There is a contingent of Catholic Stepford nunnies who, when they first heard me mention the Church, made a few attempts to recruit me. As I talked more they realized I was a wild card of a Catholic. I could break into invectives any old time, at my St. Anthony's training that taught me perfection is attainable if only I'd get my shit together and try harder, at the creepy feeling that a nun was always watching and keeping score. I enjoyed the flinch I produced in them. They were nice little mousies for whom getting dressed up meant changing the leather thong of their outsized wooden crucifix or pinning a matching enamel

Lady of Fatima cameo on their nifty navy blue suits. It was not a fair fight and the only thing I can say in my defense is that I gave them the opportunity to forgive me my sacrilege.

I'm not a heathen, and I didn't consider myself sacrilegious. I believe in God. I know what He looks like because my mother bought me a children's book on world religions when I was seven. Its endpapers featured Michelangelo's *Creation of Adam,* and that stingy curmudgeonly finger of the fierce old man was imprinted on my brain. All the cozy models in the Big Book of Alcoholics Anonymous and Vatican II sign-of-peace-think have never shaken that image. A punitive, grudging God of rules and categories of sin, who, in my myths, had not intended that I be born in the first place and, realizing His mistake, had let the consequences of me go.

I have been known to define my higher power as Prozac.

One Sunday, on a whim, I went to Mass. A mead-colored light filled the vaulted ceiling over the altar, a backdrop of virginal blue and gilt foil fleur-de-lis and papal keys reflected the light in the mellowest way. Assumption contains components of my sweeter childhood, when, perhaps, I still had a chance at not turning to the deepfreeze of food and obesity. I drowned a little in its pastel optimism, a homecoming I hadn't expected, and I found myself moved by the old automatic words of the Nicene Creed that I don't believe in but recited automatically after not having thought of it in years.

The pastor was terrific. It didn't hurt that the first sermon he preached began with the single, ominous word, "*inventory.*" It also didn't hurt that he laughed out loud at my button of New York City Mayor Rudolph Giuliani with a line across his face. "I went to school with him," he said, grabbing my hand to shake it heartily. "We'll talk."

We did talk, later, at Mother's suggestion. "If you're going to join the parish," she said, "go in and find out what he's about. Make him find out what you're about."

It was so *adult* to enroll in a parish. I had belonged to my parents' parishes for the first half of my life and shunned churches for the second. Would I be asked for a baptismal certificate? How would he know I wasn't some . . . *Lutheran,* infiltrating the papist citadel for nefarious Protestant purposes?

There is, I had always known but realized again in Father D'Angelo's office, the Church of edicts, and the Church of regular people. Father D'Angelo knows his congregants engage in all sorts of activities Rome pretends we're doing without, and he knows very well that the fate of his Church hangs on these edicts. That was the substance of our conversation, and enough I suppose to convince him I was not a Masonic spy.

One of the reasons I joined was because I saw that my presence at Mass and on the congregation's rolls mattered. It was one more instance where my actual body was needed. Further, the more people like me the congregation included—working, single, neither old nor young—the more it would attract others. It made a difference to me that I was not a three-hundred-pound bundle of despair in an empty pew.

My forehead still running with holy water on my first visit, I genuflected. For the first time since grade school I sank all the way to my knee.

A sister, a friend, a granddaughter, a member, church, the gym. What was next? Was it time to write a novel? Meet the astrophysicist with two black Labradors and a SoHo loft? I was making "next" happen by making "now" into a home.

It was these little things, I emailed to a friend who was curious to know how weight loss had changed me, that comprised the loss of—surprise! the gym had increased my tally—175 pounds. It was a hot June evening. The drone of air condition-ers batted against my open window but I didn't need to turn mine on yet. "I am writing to you in a pair of Gap khaki shorts and a black sports bra," I reported. "No one will *ever* see me this way, but I'm practicing being thin."

I was ready for my spotlight, Mr. DeMille.

10

VISIT TO THE PLANET

OF FAT

It was a soft and expansive spotlight I planned for myself, a summer of the gym, English novels, Montana in August and hiking in Glacier Park and anything else that might come up. On June 1 I weighed 161 pounds. All that nervous energy and the gym were paying off, a pound at a time. What couldn't I do, what couldn't happen?

I was particularly pleased with my life the last Monday night in late June. I'd gotten an hour on the treadmill, moseyed home for a dinner of cabbage salad with toasted sesame oil and a chilled mango while I read *Harry Potter* on my couch. A fine life, I thought as I shuffled together a manuscript I had just signed—military history, a subject I'm keen on. That night, after my hour in the gym and my cold mango, feeling floaty and freshly showered and well housed, I almost looked forward to the editing I was about to start. If only my stomach didn't feel so . . . odd.

Thirty-six hours later I threw up for the last time on a gaggle of anxious residents after they'd managed to insert a nasogastric tube in my esophagus rather than my trachea. I'd been barfing for a day and a half. My internist referred me to a surgical team at NYU Hospital, which whisked me away for IVs, an MRI, and God's revenge on human hubris, the nasogastric tube. I was in for a long haul.

The Stepfords saved my life. I called Katie after throwing up for the fourth time. She called Bridget, who insisted I go to the emergency room. When I decided, at two in the morning, that Bridget was right, I called Pam, who drove me and waited until I was escorted to a cubicle. She drove me to my internist and on to NYU a day later. "You aren't alone," Katie and Pam repeated, over and over.

I sat and shivered under a sheet, laboring to breathe around the apparatus taped to my face, already dry-mouthed and destined to another week of it. *You fucker,* I muttered in a cold vehement whisper to God. *You son of a bitch. Get me out of this. I don't want to die and I don't want to have surgery. Get* down *here: now.*

It is so not fair, I went on, rage dwindling into whining. *I ought to be thinking about Harry Potter and the gym and what movie to watch tonight.* That my oughts all happened after 5:30 P.M. gave me pause. What would I be doing right now, on a Wednesday afternoon? I'd be at my desk in that mess of an office, laboring over an abysmal manuscript, between sending out pointless magazine submissions, listening to Barbara's daughter pitch pointless novels to uninterested film scouts in banal descriptions I'd heard a hundred times. *Would I rather be here, or in the office?*

Here . . .

I would have sighed, had the NG tube allowed it. It was time to revisit last fall's resolution to get out of the office.

I would have laughed but for the same reason. It wasn't the time at all. Everything, including swallowing, would have to wait.

I'd been through this before, nasogastric hell and abdominal surgery; I knew what was coming. Worse, I'd brought it on myself. My intestines were strangled in scarring from the surgery twelve years earlier to remove my gall bladder and a thirty-six-pound ovarian cyst, malfunctioning because of the food I ate and the hormonal imbalances that resulted from my obesity. I was face-to-face with the most serious consequences of what I had done to my body, had fought for two and a half years to undo, or pretend away.

The gods of the Planet of Fat were as restless to restake their claim as my escorts on the Planet of Girls were to keep me in their ranks. Katie was on the phone with surgery every hour until I was wheeled into ICU, relaying updates to my parents and making sure Dennis was at my bedside when I woke up to the ventilator. "I thought you'd want to know your wallet is safe," he said, and smoothed my hair.

Still, the Home Planet was checking in, calling collect.

Perhaps I knew that best when I resurfaced from an afternoon morphine nap to see Barbara sitting in the chair at the foot of my bed. Quickly, I rationalized: nasogastric tube siphoning off bile, catheter, IV, morphine clicker going like mad, a drain drizzling more brown guck from my belly. Convincing enough?

"I'm sorry I'm not at work," I said, half ironically, half cringingly. This had to be the best excuse I'd ever pulled off.

"Oh, Frahncees."

She gave me a purple stone engraved with the word "health" and didn't stay long. I liked that stone. It cupped coolly in my left hand, matching the morphine drip that lay in my right palm. Later I heard of her concern about the morphine. My body had to be fed and drained from orifices natural and unnatural but it was the painkillers that she fretted over? It held a perfect illogic.

What ye put up with, so shall ye have. I'd given twelve years to that office and reaped a cold smooth stone. I'd put two years into making my body healthier and still it was the playground of capricious dark angels.

After a week I was liberated from most of the tubes and Katie smuggled miso soup to me. "You need live foods, Frances. Tofu and yogurt. We need to get good bacteria in your intestines again. I looked it up on the 'net." Tracy hustled in the morning I was released, cleared the paperwork with professional speed, and drove me home. I wept with weakness and gratitude when she propped me up for my first shower in weeks, too shaky to do it alone or be embarrassed as she toweled me off and rubbed lotion on my back. She'd cleaned my apartment and done the laundry, and came by every few days to change my bandages, a task that frightened me.

What didn't the Stepfords do? Katie marshaled them all. Nora stayed until I was ready to fall asleep at night after a scary bout of fevers. Katie cooked and packaged premeasured meals, and Pam took me for drives, a much-needed break from the Bat Cave; Amy brought me cash to pay for antibiotics.

Thank God I'd bought a bed.

"Stand up straight," my father advised, "or you'll grow back funny. And don't expect your brain to work."

He was right. Nothing worked. I was muzzy from anesthesia and morphine, and I looked blankly at the work Barbara forwarded to me at home, unable to make what should have been instinctive decisions. My email was full with clients wanting to know what was going on with their submissions.

In the two weeks I spent in Brooklyn, my body became the magician's hat of some masterful jokesters. I was weak as a kitten, dismayed that I couldn't even shut my window. My newly liberated bowels were unpredictable, and I wobbled as each day I ventured farther away from the front door.

My frailty and keen need for lots of space around my stomach widened the gulf for someone who was already straddling two bodies: one fat, the other adjusting to being normal. A few weeks earlier I had still wondered if I stepped into that crowded elevator, would everyone feel invaded, only to remind myself I took up no more room than anyone else who needed to get to the eleventh floor. If I twisted to answer the phone while folding laundry, would my precarious sense of balance capsize me into the closet door? (I broke a toe in that way.) If I got distracted by garlic smells coming from Lichee Nut on Montague Street, would I trip on a sidewalk crack? (I broke my face and glasses that way.) On any day in my new body, I found my depth perception tenuous, newly aware of the world because the effort of moving around in it was lost. It was as colorful and inviting as a buffet, putting me in a shaky state of scattered alertness, often magnified by actual hunger.

Now I really was shaky and addled. My stomach was once again the center of my physical universe. People crowded too close to it, I was prone to sudden incontinence. These were the physical sensations, magnified, of the early days of weight loss when my digestive tract was adjusting to my radical change in diet and I was accompanied, every minute, by the 313 pounds I was lumbering to change. The triumph of bending over to tie my shoelaces was lost. Bandaged and sore, I found my old size 44 bloomer underwear. I was wearing elastic or drawstring pants from summers long past, my Gap shorts and jeans forgotten. Continuing slight fevers made me as clammy and reactive to the summer heat wave as my obesity had.

But I wasn't obese. Two weeks of IVs had their effect. Dennis was dying to know the truth of it and had searched out a scale on the hospital ward: 155 pounds. Less, at last, than he weighed at six feet one.

The surgery compromised my digestion and capacity, necessitating changes in my food plan. Fruit in midmorning and afternoon, fewer vegetables, well cooked, more carbohydrates, cranberry juice to combat a bladder infection my father assured me was typical from catheters. Katie and Bridget cobbled this plan together, but it boggled me after two years of rigorously boundaried and defined habits.

My stomach was controlling my life again, and I was voracious. Well stocked with Katie's steamed yams and baked salmon, all I wanted to do was eat; surrounded by the Stepfords, my inquisitive appetite felt furtive and dirty. Food had new glamour to my deprived palate, it broke up the tedium of watching the hundred-year-long A&E *Pride and Prejudice. It was the wrong ten pounds,* I told myself as I ordered tandoori chicken with Katie's cautious OK. *I need* live *food,* I justified as I bought brie. These are foods that fit our criteria of no sugar and no flour but they are seductive, entrancing, dangerous.

The gods of the Planet of Fat—pissed off, maybe, at everything I'd been doing right—had more pranks in their bag of tricks. In a day, the wrong ten pounds turned into the wrong *twenty* pounds gained as my ankles swelled and the scale rocketed to 174 pounds. Nineteen pounds in a night? I wept to Katie, to my father. I wasn't eating *that* much. Steroids, Daddy speculated. They might have administered steroids during surgery. "You come home and we'll get you on hydrochlorothiazide," he said comfortably, and I longed, all 174 puffed pounds of me, to be beamed to the east shore of Flathead Lake, under my daddy's care, familiar in his own meld of indifference and automatic expertise. My surgeon was noncommittal and unconcerned as he removed the last of the stitches. "Go home to your family," he agreed. "You need rest and fresh air."

If my life is in New York, and my heart in Venice, my soul belongs to Flathead. I wanted it like some necessary nutrient—sweet air, eleven o'clock dusks, dew, the songs of the lake mildly lapping the shore, swallows nesting. I wanted not to be in charge of my weakness anymore, to hand it to my daddy and his old skills and sure touch.

It turned out that New York's air was a lot fresher than Montana's. Flathead, like the rest of the state, was on fire that summer, the mountains spuming smoke and ashes, volcanic rather than glacial. I woke every morning to the pall of forests burning around the Flathead Valley, the west shore, five miles away, often invisible. We watched the mountain our orchard sits at the base of for rogue lightning strikes that would have the entire bay scuttling.

Each morning, in addition to the acrid haze that was so thick that Missoula, ninety miles south, had its streetlights on all day, I woke to the smell of my father's elaborate breakfasts and discussions of the next meal. Meals occupy a huge portion of retirees' conversation, and cooking had always been a favorite topic with my parents. "I'm not hungry after that big breakfast," Dad would say early in the afternoon. "I'll just have crackers and cheese," followed by a handful of my favorite oatmeal cookies and comments on my lunch.

"Sure is a lot of—what is that? cauliflower?—you're eating there." Mom peered into my mixing bowl. "How much is that? You eat so *much* . . ."

This was my fifth visit to them on my food plan. I spread my hands, a gesture of bratty impatience that invited a look-see at the body that took up half the space it used to.

Or maybe not half the size. Dad's water pills had worked—for four pounds. I was steadyish at around 170 pounds. I stood on their scale with a hundred ish-reasons. My stomach was still so swollen I had to buy drawstring shorts at Target, a size 20.

Altitude. Doesn't altitude add a couple of pounds?

It wasn't my scale. It was probably a few pounds off.

I wasn't going to the gym, wasn't walking farther than across the highway and down the hill to the lake. I was not yet allowed to swim. My time in the water was spent on a giant inner tube reading Smollett. To an inveterate pedestrian, sevenish pounds would be easy. It would all come off as soon as I got back to commuting.

It was only seven pounds, or around seven pounds. Around two, if I considered that I'd spent quite content months the fall before at 168.

I continued to spread my hands to Mom's offers of peaches or cantaloupe an hour after lunch. "No thanks," I said in reminding her, a little guiltily, of my rules around food. Would she ever get it? Yes, I eat an embarrassing amount of vegetables. No, I don't snack, even on fruit.

Or not much. It was five weeks of being within fifteen feet of that kitchen. Sometimes I took a handful of cherries while we played cards. Hadn't I been having a midafternoon fruit a few weeks ago?

Previous visits to Montana had been easier because my parents have a guest house. My niece and grandniece, Lisa and Sophie, were staying there as Lisa's divorce was finalized. Added to the always plentiful kitchen my parents kept was their desire to feed two temperamental guests. "Grandma." Sophie batted her eyes at my mother at least twice a week. "Will you make me a *pie*?" The next afternoon there would be *two* pies, my mother's and my father's, vying for "best pie in the toddler class." Sophie would have two bites and skip off to her coloring books and I, cooped up in a small house with an unending cycle of meals going on around me, would be left at the table to watch ice cream melt into the maroon pool of cherries or apple slices winking with cinnamon or peaches oozing from a lard crust.

And still the gods had malice to spare. One night I staggered into the living room after an hour's sleep, drenched in sweat. My father was still up, reading; he looked at me quizzically.

"Do I have a fever?" I asked, and bent down to his rough-palmed, old knowledge.

"No."

"I'm wet through." I pulled my nightshirt out and, sure enough, it clung with damp resistance. "What the hell is *this*?"

"How old are you, kid?"

"Forty-three."

He humphed and shook his magazine back into place. "You're down one battery and you're forty-three," he said matter-of-factly, referring to the ovary I had lost ten years before. "It's called night sweats. It's called menopause."

Menopause. A lot of friends my age had kids just out of diapers and I was starting menopause.

A few nights later I came staggering out to my father again, this time with a dull pain that was slowly tying my gut in knots. I sat down and took a few cautious breaths.

"Problems?" he asked, this time in a voice that conveyed his recognition of something bad. All of us in the family know that voice and it scares us. Dad takes only the serious things seriously.

"I might have to go to the hospital."

I described the funny thud I'd felt earlier and ignored, mounting now into something pushing bluntly, a hammer-headed alien ready to strike.

"It's like that night," I panted, and leaned back in the chair as close to a 180-degree angle as I could muster. "Before I started throwing up. Like I gotta barf a basketball. Something big."

"Let's wait and see if you do," he said. "Go lie down again and see if you feel better. If you don't, wake me up. We'll get you to Polson. We'll call Jesse in the morning."

It subsided, but not completely and not until I saw Jesse, who prescribed something.

"What are you eating?" Katie asked when I told her about this new infusion of pain. I'd reverted to raw vegetables in a half-assed attempt to take off the two or seven or ten or fifteen pounds—I didn't want to know. "Stick to what we were doing before. I don't think you can handle the raw vegetables, and certainly not sixteen ounces of them."

This was license for the Home Planet gods to mutter sneaky invitations. Why not a fruit at midmorning? Those green beans looked skimpy, have more potato. I was listless and stale and growing angrier and lonelier by the day. Everything I liked was in smithereens—no email, no list of things to do, no gossip, a two-hour time difference between me and the Stepfords that made contact expensive and unlikely, and what was there to say? The phrase "food plan" felt fake and stupid three thousand miles out of context. I didn't feel thin with my bloomer under-wear and drawstring shorts. I had no *news* whatsoever. My par-ents and I had said everything of consequence in the first day of my return, if not years before, and I squirmed to find something fresh to talk about. Blue Bay is twenty minutes from the nearest grocery store, ninety minutes from Missoula with its movies and what few friends I had left there. If friends in New York asked what was going on, what I was doing, all I could tell them was that the mountains were on fire and I was reading eighteenth-century novels. What response could they give? "I've seen the news. It looks terrible." Or "Oh. How nice."

Wheel of Fortune threatened to induce psychosis. When Mom convinced me to watch with her I would mutter, "Bankrupt, bankrupt," with increasing volume throughout the endless half hour.

I seethed, read, and got tan.

Because I couldn't swim and the beach I used was reached by a steep rocky path with Oregon grapes for handholds, I was hanging out on the Warrens' lakefront, a neat-as-a-pin concrete embankment and deck, outlined in dazzling impatiens and pansies, with ladders to the water. Bill and Jan Warren are good friends. They kept an eye on my parents' house eight months of the year, hosted terrific parties, shared their bumper crops of zucchini and their chaise lounges. I got tan for the first time in a dozen years, roasting in the fire-hazy sun until my whole body called for the stunning cold of the lake. I evolved a slow-motion maneuver to sidle down a ladder and onto my inner tube without straining my stomach. Their deck was the one place I could get away from my parents' two-bedroom house, but I did not get away from the omnipresence of food.

At the end of the afternoon, after working in their orchard through another broiling day of fires, the Warrens meandered down to the deck, dove in the lake, and came up for cocktails. I didn't imbibe, but I did partake—the ubiquitous cherries, peanuts, home-smoked lake trout, the crudités and guacamole with extra cayenne and cilantro. I had justifications—I'd be eating dinner in an hour and this was on my food plan; I'd reduce my protein; the cold of the lake would freeze it off; I'd missed lunch.

As ye eat so shall ye reap.

It's not so much that I gained weight. I stayed around the 174 pounds I arrived at, although I could no longer claim it was a water weight phantom. I was, moment by moment, cherry by cantaloupe ball, out of control. By not being square with my knowledge of how I and food coexist, I was not square with myself. Every day I let something creep in. If it wasn't sugar or flour, it was messy and queasy, and I got nastier and nastier at cheering for *Wheel of Fortune* bankruptcies. And still my food made me stick out. "*When* can you drink again?" Jan asked as she poured herself a glass of wine. "These cookies are really good. You can have *one*, can't you?" I eyed it all with envy and no, I could not have one. One would never suffice.

The close quarters of my parents' house and my boredom crested when my brother and his family came up for the weekend. Now it was seven people in a small house, televisions on upstairs and down, and perpetual eating. I turned sullen, then mean, refusing to speak and slapping off my sister-in-law's sympathetic hug as I was toiling to assemble vegetables while she put spaghetti on the table. I hated them and I hated myself. I had to get away and there was no place to go. There wasn't even a telephone I could use that wasn't in an occupied room. I volunteered to do the dishes alone and lapped at the spaghetti sauce. A few days later, my parents announced they'd had lunch after their golf game and weren't hungry. "I need the car keys," I huffed. "I'll have to drive into Polson to get food *I* can eat." I drove seventy miles an hour along the sharp curves and narrow highway to Polson, came home, and made the biggest bowl of oatmeal in the world, and then another, and then another.

Which I ate in my room with the door closed.

Woozy on a hot August evening, I shoved the dish under my bed. So. Here I was. Furtively creeping out to snatch food to gobble alone in my room. Eating in the bed I'd eaten in for seventeen years. I would sleep badly and hotly through the night, wake to the crusty bowl under the bed and my fidgetiness at my parents, myself, the weeks still to be endured that would contain the same choler. *Very nice, Frances.* Or I could go wash the bowl, cop to what I'd done. I heaved myself into the kitchen and washed the bowl, went into the air-conditioned dining room and started shuffling cards.

"I ate," I said to my mother as she fetched the penny jars for spite and malice.

"I thought so," she answered.

"I fucked up."

"I'm sorry it's so hard on you, honey."

"I'm sorry, too."

The next morning I called Katie and told her what I'd done. I was scared. I'd never done anything like this—would she drop me? Would she scold me? I gabbled about how torturous things were, knowing it sounded lame, until she cut in.

"Frances. Frances. Of *course* you ate. You're a compulsive overeater. You ate. Nothing wrong or weird about it. Now you have to stop."

Such a simple statement, such grace in the allowance. When it came to food, I would always be purple-skinned with webbed feet. I'd had a colossal tantrum, triggered by my parents' mistake in not picking up chicken and yogurt, the lack of privacy, isolation from the Stepfords. I was a compulsive overeater; I ate. My food journal would always open to that day because I taped in a postcard of a winter Flathead and wrote below it, "I feel fragile as new ice."

I improved. My food improved but it wasn't perfect. I was allowed to swim, and I felt stronger. I saw friends in Missoula who didn't recognize me as I walked toward them in front of the restaurant. It felt good to say to myself, *I'm meeting friends for lunch,* made me feel like a friend. The weeks were funneling toward my return to New York and I began to appreciate being at Flathead, a treasure chest of colors: teal lake, sun-bleached sky, long forest-fired sunsets. I slept late and deeply for knowing the time was finite, read happily rather than desperate for distraction, knowing that in a few weeks I'd be back to manuscripts. I sat out at night to watch the sunsets and the meteors and the bats. These were the things I wanted to remember.

Near the end of my stay, now as miserable at the thought of

Barbara as I had been at being stranded in Montana, I took up permanent residence on the Warrens' deck, compelled to get as tan as possible in compensation for the weight I'd gained. Tanning was not easy for me. I burned bright red wherever I hadn't gotten half-hour applications of no. 30 sunblock. I let the Warrens know I could be ignored—they had visitors and I had books to read—but they invited me into the forty-eight-hour party. Because the tan was the thing and we were all middle aged, I spent two days in my swimming suit and nothing else— no T-shirt to hide my sagging arms, no towel wrapped Bali style around my venous lumpy thighs. It was my body in a black Speedo, with acres of sun, a reflecting lake, and a convivial group that included a buff divorced man my age named Rick. Rick and I sat on the concrete wall for a few minutes here and there, chatting about not much, as I did with everyone in those two days. I watched him from behind my sunglasses, his belly concave, brown, and muscled in loose cutoffs that gapped interestingly, blond hair he flopped off his forehead, runner's legs. My arms jiggled when I reached for seltzer and I felt frowsy without a recent color job or Ella's waxing. I didn't care. I'd never see him again and I turned silly as a teenager when Jan pulled me aside.

"Rick thinks you're cute."

"I think he's cute."

"He was askin' about you. 'Who's *that*? Is she single?' I told him you're Doc Kuffel's daughter, that you're leaving in ten days and he shouldn't get any ideas."

"Those are good questions, right?"

"*Don't* sleep with him! He's one of our best friends but he's a mess."

"Don't worry. I'd have to know his middle name first. But he said I'm cute, right?" I squealed in a whisper.

Jan looked at me warningly, then grinned. There I was, Speedo, my long brown leggy legs, my eyes bluer for my tan, and my face exposed with my wet hair slicked back. I looked like somebody who, if she wanted to have sex with a Rick, would.

Could.

Might.

I didn't know it, but I'd just learned the First Law of Men. If a man asks if you're available he's hoping you are.

Even if your arms have wings and the scale and your waistbands are scolding you. Even if his interest lasted the time it took to ask and meant nothing more than the bat of a butterfly's wings in Hong Kong.

Then again, a butterfly sneezes in China and rocks the molecules that brew the hurricane that flattens Curaçao.

Hmm, I thought. *Information. Rick, who probably goes for big-boobed, big-haired frosted blondes with blue and pink eye shadow and ass-splitting stone-washed jeans, red Tony Lamas, and jaw-bone-length feathered earrings. And yet he wondered about the availability of my very visible and imperfect body.*

I smiled slyly, savoring it and saving it for the intangible September that was rushing toward me. A butterfly had sneezed; I had a beat of hope.

11

S.O.S.

I continued to itch with dissatisfaction when I returned to New York. Sooner or later it would be time to start putting in a full day's work. I couldn't go on alluding to my stomach and telling Barbara, "Rush hour frightens me," without lying about the prognosis Dr. Chang had given me. But an eight-hour day in that office? Jesus, Mary, and Joseph, it was against all humanity.

I was headed to the office, the office, the office. Thirteen pounds heavier than three months earlier.

Hadn't I gone through this rebellion a year ago? I was going around the same damn mountain again.

Katie, I learned in our morning phone calls, had issues.

"My therapist thinks I'm too rigid about food," she said more than once when I called in my day's food that October. "I'm beginning to think she's right. Spontaneity is an issue for me. We're really digging into issues. Food, body, work. You should think about therapy, Frances."

"Mm-hm," I allowed tepidly. I couldn't see how it applied to me. My food issues were apparent: let me eat the way I wanted and I'd be 338 pounds faster than you could say large-with-extra-cheese, which pretty much covered the subject of my body issues as well. Better not to think about either.

I had no patience for issues when I had an arsenal of facts. I couldn't settle down to my job, couldn't look at Barbara or talk to my clients. I couldn't lose that seven—or thirteen—pounds. Maybe Katie was content with talk-talk-talk, but the *fact* was that both of us were wearing clothes that the year before had been form-fitting and now cut into our flesh. I couldn't button the blazer of the suit Mom bought me a year ago. Well, I countered, you're not really supposed to button it. Had I been able to the year before? I couldn't quite remember.

"Barbara looked at me funny yesterday," I reported to Katie morning after chilly morning. "Barbara didn't believe I made those magazine submissions until I produced the complete documentation," I sulked. "Barbara"—be praised!—"complimented me on a sale." Barbara, Barbara, Barbara.

Weighing an apple denied Katie freedom, she reported to me morning after chilly morning. Weighing an apple showed lack of trust in her body's metabolism and her own judgment. Weighing an apple was a pain in the ass. Weighing, weighing, weighing.

We were immolating, Katie and I. She was trying to put out the fire. I was walking combustibility.

"You need to get into therapy," she said bluntly at last. The Halloween witches had given way to harvest paraphernalia on the neighborhood stoops and she'd listened to my soaking misery long enough. Sponsoring my rage was not her job. "Promise you'll make an appointment."

"I can't afford it," I said glumly.

"Call your insurance company and ask if it's covered."

The next morning. "Did you call?"

"No. I didn't have time. Barbara was in and—"

"Call. Take one action."

My insurance company gave me a choice of categories: therapists, and addiction therapists.

"A regular therapist," I answered, and then changed my mind. "An addiction therapist."

"Do you have a drinking or drug problem?" the representative asked.

"No."

"But you want an addiction therapist."

"Do you consider Pop-Tarts an addiction?" I asked. She laughed. "I'm in recovery for food addiction."

"Really?" she said. "Have you lost weight?"

"Yeah," I said, switching into my story. "A hundred and seventy-five pounds." I was fudging the truth, clinging to last spring's best-case scenario.

"I need to lose fifty," she confided. Everyone who needs to lose a hundred pounds says they need to lose fifty.

She asked where I wanted to find a therapist, and quickly narrowed it to a tight radius within the office. I stopped her after three names and numbers. My theory of conveniences had been tested again; I had no excuses. An hour later I had an interview set up for the next day.

Take one right action. The next will reveal itself.

I did my shtick for Dr. Miller—the 170 . . . well, 150 pounds, how I'd never gotten comfortable in this body, my rage at no parade in my honor, how surgery had interrupted my beloved routines, how work was destroying my peace of mind.

"Tell me about your family," she responded in her broad

Manhattan accent. I shifted into family shtick. I'd had a hundred years of therapy. It had kept me together with Scotch tape and rubber bands in college while we didn't talk about my weight. I forged back in time: adoption, skanky oldest brother whose corpse I was glad to see thirteen years ago, parents not around much, a childhood of self-loathing that manifested in my girth or my girth that trained me in self-loathing. As I recited I wondered if I could get help from this Dr. Miller. She was a Zaftig, making this small office home in small touches—a not overwhelming cat motif, tulips—unimpressed at my achievement, quintessentially New York. She told me later that when she went to graduate school, she took boxes of Maybelline with her because she didn't think they had mascara in the Midwest. Would she understand what it means to me to be (OK, not thin, not anymore) inhabiting a body no longer abnormal? To be a Montana girl in New York? To be tolerated but not liked for forty hours a week? She didn't strike me as one who would tolerate mere tolerance.

"Give me an example of the dynamic with your boss," Dr. Miller said. I thought back over the years of petty humiliations.

"The air conditioners," I decided. "They weren't working, so Mr. Kazin—we call Barbara, Barbara, but her husband is always Mr. Kazin; he has no job that anyone can see, so he does all our computers and wiring and stuff, and nothing works very long or the way it's supposed to—anyway, Mr. Kazin came in and took the air conditioners apart. When he realized he couldn't fix them he left. They were in a million pieces all over Barbara's office. She came back from lunch and asked what had happened. I told her Mr. Kazin had tried to fix them but couldn't and left them that way. 'Well, put them back together, Frahncees, my husband is *not* a janitor, you know.' "

"And you've been there *twelve years*? Why don't you leave?"

Was she nuts? Had her clients infected her with their many insanities, hour after hour of listening to Upper East Side kvetching?

"I don't know how to *do* anything."

"Fran, come on! I'm sure there's *something* you can do."

"Yeah? Who would want me?"

"What you're really saying is that your parents, or Barbara, could—what?—take you back to the dog pound if they decide they don't like you? Get a refund?"

"Barbara can fire me," I maintained. "She's threatened to."

"You've got to get out."

Tense as a cast iron skillet on full flame, my morning calls to Katie were full of Dr. Miller and my inaction. My reluctance to leave my job wasn't just lack of confidence, it was also the eerie feeling that Barbara and I had been together longer than twelve years, that there was some karmic thing that had to be worked out. Maybe the soul of my third-grade nun, Sister Mary Francesca, had migrated into Barbara.

"I turn to Silly Putty with Barbara," remembering the demon of St. Anthony's who was determined to be displeased by all but a few good girls of whom I was too messy to be counted among. "I want to learn how to stop turning to Silly Putty. Barbara seems like a chance to do that. Isn't therapy about changing yourself so you can change your life? Dr. Miller says sometimes you have to change your life, that your 'self' will catch up eventually. I'm not sure she's right."

"Do an inventory on your relationship with Barbara," Katie said. "Use the Big Book format and see what *you* come up with."

I took out my copy of *Alcoholics Anonymous*, the bible of all twelve-step programs, and studied the fourth step: "Made a searching and fearless moral inventory of ourselves." I bought a $1.59 notebook and ruled out three columns with the Big Book's headings: "Resentment," "How it affects me," and "My character defect."

I began with the air conditioners. The effect of that comment was that I felt *I* was a janitor. *I*, Frances Kuffel, a doctor's daughter with a master's degree who could quote John Berryman and . . . and—I sputtered—and whose vanity had been pricked with dead accuracy.

Pride. The first of the seven deadly sins.

It didn't matter, according to the Big Book, how I'd been treated. It was the defect of character that needed improvement.

Just ducky, I thought. *Another "I am personally responsible for the agony of Christ" moment.*

"So," I balked to Katie the next morning, "this fourth step thing turns everything into my fault? Is that how this works?"

"Keep at it," she said, so I did.

The inventory grew into two pages of crabbed handwriting documenting Barbara's collisions with my pride, ambition, need for approval, fear, selfishness about my time and energy. The self-accusation that I had no real job skills turned nastier with each addition to the list of my faults. I seemed to be comprised of faults.

"How many items are on your list?" the Good Doctor Miller asked when I told her about my newest project.

"Thirty-six so far, in no particular order."

"You can stop, Fran. You've proved your point. You've got to get out."

And so it went. Until one day I was having lunch with an editor from St. Martin's, eating perfectly delicious roast chicken and mashed potatoes as I described a kooky mystery I represented, and half a crown fell away. It was there, it was not there. I had swallowed a sizable wad of tooth with my haricots verts.

I'd never paid for my own dental work, never gone to a dentist in New York.

"Is this my fault, too?" I asked my father. "Did I destroy my teeth with sugar?"

"Who knows?" he said. "A crown'll run you, oh, a good seven hundred dollars."

Or how about ten thousand? I had as much access to one sum as the other. It didn't matter who would want me. I had to get another job.

But what? How? It had been over a decade since I'd picked up the help-wanted ads and lied about how fast I could type.

At least the crown gave me one more excuse for being out of the office. I milked it for more than it was worth.

"Frahncees," Barbara intoned. "It's time for you to settle down. It's been four months since you were in the hospital, and the dentist cawn't take this much time."

She was right but I snapped. She made her own hours—if only I could, too. If only I had a little time. Maybe I could write something I could sell. A few hours stood between me and a full set of teeth.

"I can't afford this crown," I said with narrowed eyes. "The only way I can pay for it is if I can pull something else together. I'd like to have Friday afternoons off to write."

She gave me a long look, measuring my seriousness. I was neither sniveling nor self-justifying.

"I'll have to think about that." A few days later she set up a lunch with me. On a Friday. I began to think hard.

Maybe I'd leave publishing altogether. I thought of leaving a nine-hour day without homework, going home to read actual books, hit the gym, sit at my computer. Maybe I could get a

marketing job at Ralph Lauren—who better than I to speak for
the clothes?

"Read *What Color Is Your Parachute?*" Katie advised. "It
helped me a lot when I had to change jobs. It focused me."

"Get your hair colored. You need to look your best for interviews," the Good Doctor Miller said.

I was talking computer courses and she was talking Clairol?
I groaned. She ignored me. Initially, my resistance had amused
her. She would roll her eyes and plow through my noise to make
a point. Sometimes it was an insight out of Alice Miller or *The
North American Field Guide to Personality Disorders*; sometimes it was hair color or a restaurant tip.

"You should go to the Five O'Clock Club," she added, and
wrote down a phone number for a group that met to talk about
changing careers.

Instead, I begged books from editor friends—*Brutal Bosses
and Their Prey, When Smart People Work for Dumb Bosses,
The Bully at Work*—and piled them conspicuously on my office
desk.

I was early for lunch, already seated and reading the latest novel
by an ex-client who had left Barbara at the time he was finishing this book.

It was a thick, hardcover glossy book. I carried nothing else
with me.

Passive aggression. It has its moments.

She had no surprises. My earnings did not justify an afternoon off. She condemned the way I worked with magazines.
Yada-yada-yada. Then the cautious caveat that provoked a response from me at last.

"I want you to know, Frahncees, I . . . respect . . . what you've . . . *done*." She looked at me meaningfully.

She meant the weight. Not the eighty-odd books I'd sold but my weight loss.

"And I want you to know I went through your surgery *with* you. But I want you to get your numbers up."

I was exceedingly proud of my weight loss, but it was not what I wanted my boss to respect me for. I wanted my earnings to increase as well. After all, if I could sell $850,001 worth of manuscripts in a year, I'd get a thirty-three-cent bonus.

But she jolly well had *not* gone through surgery with me.

Staying in the agency was one more form of obesity, a refusal to take responsibility for myself, an outward sign of how little I thought I deserved from people and how much I still depended on external definitions—food or clothing labels or opinions—of myself.

I put my fork down with a decided *clack* on the plate. It had the effect of forming the line I was about to draw. "I want you to know I will be looking for other employment," I said. "I don't know when I will leave, but I will leave."

Barbara gave me her hundred-yard stare, daring me to say the next incriminating thing. I stared back. I meant it. We had no terms to negotiate and I wasn't giving in. I could see her make her decision in favor of a certain kind gracefulness.

"You can accomplish anything you want to do, Frahncees, you've shown that."

So it still came down to the weight. I did that, therefore I can do—what?

I went back to the office and stripped all the cartoons and junk I'd amassed over the years, and sorted books into two piles: one to take home, one to donate to the library. Barbara blinked at the bare bulletin board and shelves, the absence of any occupancy except for *The Bully at Work* at my right hand, in fluorescent orange.

"Oh," she said, and stopped right there.

"I want to be ready," I said, and turned back to my computer.

Take an action. I called a publishing employment agency and made an appointment as a birthday present to myself. The representative was flummoxed by my résumé—an agent? They placed assistants in agencies, of course, but what, exactly, does an agent *do?*

I explained I didn't want to be an agent anymore, I wanted to do anything else if it paid forty thousand dollars a year.

The recruiter slid my résumé into a folder and said she'd be in touch. She was, a week later. She had a friend. Her friend had written a children's book. She wondered if I might represent it. I did not return the call.

I walked into the Christmas season with the sullen, angry part of myself accounted for and articulated. Therapy and a fourth-step inventory had given words to an ugly side of me, but putting it into words allowed me to feel sorry for that ugly alien stewing within. She had been scolded, punished, silenced, and ignored, and she'd mollified her resentment at such treatment with food. Deprived of food, she'd gotten angrier yet. Maybe in the new year I'd get to trot out the Girl. Sorting out all that muck got me back to the basics. I needed a crown. I had to make a living.

On a sleeting morning in early January, the recruiter from the publishing agency left me another message. This time, it said, it was not about a friend's book.

"Can you negotiate contracts?" she asked when I called back.

"Uh, yeah, it's sort of what an agent *does*." I rolled my eyes.

"Can you read a royalty statement? Do you have a slate of editorial contacts? Do you have a client base of your own? Have you spoken at conferences?"

Yes, yes, yes, yes. "What is this job, anyway?" I interrupted.

A literary agent was looking for an executive vice president. The recruiter who had coolly dismissed my prospects was now Ms. Eager Beaver. This was a hell of a lot more lucrative than the entry-level positions she specialized in.

"Can I ask who this agent is?" When she told me, I laughed. I'd dealt with her at arm's length over business before. High-strung, I remembered. Rather prone to hysterics under pressure. Executive vice president for her? It was such a long shot that I laughed again and responded, "Oh, I know Alix. Say hi for me. Wish her luck!"

An hour later, an interview had been arranged.

I walked into her offices overlooking Central Park, put my hand out to a petite shimmering woman, and said, "Hello, I'm Frances Kuffel."

"Of course," she said smoothly. "We know each other from the Association of Authors' Representatives. Come in and give me your coat."

Barbara would have gestured vaguely, waiting either for an underling to take the coat or for the guest to fumble in the closet. Everything was already different.

"Why do you want to leave Barbara's agency?" she asked as I handed her a fresh copy of my résumé on good stock paper.

I thought a moment before responding. "Things have changed radically, even catastrophically, for me. I need a change of employment as well. I don't know if I want to be an agent at all."

"Oh?"

"There are some editorial options I'm pursuing. Or maybe I want to leave the business. I don't know."

I looked down at my lap. I was wearing a dark gray suit and the skirt hiked up when I sat. My legs were crossed and my knees, no matter how fucked up my food and my weight felt—my knees were so *thin*.

That's what I remember most about the interview, that and the headlights of traffic winkling among the winter-bare trees of Central Park West far beneath us.

The following Tuesday I was back in Alix's office going over my client list with a fine-tooth comb. She explained aspects of my position.

"I am offering you this job," she said after two hours.

"You don't have to," I answered. The initial interview had provoked me to make an organized round of phone calls to publishers and editors-in-chief asking if they had editorial positions open. I hadn't seriously considered that a decision would be demanded within eight days of what she had told me was her first interview. "We can continue this romance for a while."

"I am offering you the job. I will have a package for you after the weekend."

"I have some leads I'm pursuing," I gulped. "I'll try to be as quick as possible about them but I can't say yes until I've spoken to some other people."

She glared at me. It was a nice glare, the fierceness of being stalked by a zoo gatherer rather than a trophy hunter. "I'll be in touch with the employment agency," she announced. "Next week. Be ready to make your decision."

Three weeks later I sat in her office trying to absorb the employment contract Alix presented me. My hands were cold and shaking at the immediate prospect the job entailed—her two assistants had quit and we had to hire a staff and train them to do things I didn't yet know how to do. *Oh, what the heck,* I thought, and signed it. Alix countersigned with a flourish worthy of Times Square.

"Remind me," I said as I placed my copy in a folder and prepared to take her dictation for the two job openings, "in six months when I know how to do this job, that I have to get a boyfriend. I've never had one and I want one."

"It can't be six months," she answered gaily.

Maybe neither of us knew whether she was saying it couldn't be six months of learning the job or six months of waiting to find something like love.

"This is the hardest winter I've ever survived," I told Dr. Miller a few weeks after starting my new job, after beginning to lose weight at last.

"Wait until you start dating," she said dryly.

"Dating." I laughed. "What's so hard about dating?"

"That's an interesting reaction."

I shrugged. "Dating will be men dismissing me because I'm not their type or not pretty enough or something. This is a *job.* I got hired because of who *I* am. It's harder to be dismissed because I'm not smart than because I'm not pretty."

"OK, Fran." She sighed the sigh of *Have it your way*—I *don't want to be the one to tell you that Santa Claus doesn't exist.*

"Whatever," I said. Didn't she know me well enough to understand that I'd staked my whole life on being smart? "I have lots of practice at not being pretty enough or thin enough. Dating isn't personal, not like . . ."

But I couldn't finish the sentence. Somewhere in the attic of my brain, I stumbled over the fact that my life had become entirely personal. I'd been hired not for my typing but for my talent, taste, skills, record. Was that the entire package of me, or was there more, something only men could answer? The alien had finished the empirical portion of her GSATs of girlhood. Now it was time to show how I would use it.

12

ALIEN VISITORS

FROM THE PLANET OF MEN

More mornings than not, Pam drove me absolutely batshit.

Pam had now lost a hundred pounds. She continued, however, to live in the eye of a hurricane.

"I'm gonna go back to bed as soon as I move the car," she said through the crackle of her cell phone. Alternate side of the street parking was in effect and she was shivering in her car, waiting for a spot. She wouldn't be eating until at least ten. I did not approve. "Breakfast'll be a third-cup rice cereal, two ounces of soy cheese, and—I don't know what's ripe."

Rice gruel and fake cheese? I prefer heartier fare. Steel-cut oats, brown rice, a steamed yam. How could she not know what fruit was ripe? How much advance planning does that take, exactly?

"Bass-tahd!" she screeched in her Queens accent. Parking mornings could turn Tourette with no warning. "Shit! He took up two whole spaces. Damn. *Hey, pull up, whydontcha?* Mutha-fucka," she muttered darkly.

We hadn't even gotten to lunch yet.

I owed Pam, and not just because she took me to the hospital at three in the morning. She lived out loud and extravagantly, like Mimi in *La Bohème*. Grudgingly at times, I had to love her hearty laugh and the easy clarion exuberance with which she made friends. Whereas I certainly bragged about my pounds lost, they were Girl Scout badges, assignments rather than celebrations. Pam knew how to celebrate. I listened to her talk about being able to wipe herself while still sitting on the toilet for the first time in years, to her teary arrival at size 20 jeans, and I envied her astonishment at her own blond Nordic beauty that evolved with each pound lost. She called the monthly good news the "happy dance."

Pam was a tour de force when it came to men.

While having occasional afternoon trysts with a married man, she was in love with Sam who lived in New Jersey and was paying for his divorce by working three jobs and seeing his kids on weekends.

"Can we separate these guys and take a look at them individually?" I interrupted her compilation tape of love in the afternoon. "One is married, the other doesn't have time to see you. There's something wrong with this picture. Have you thought about dating a single man with one job?"

"That's Nick. I'm spending the weekend with him."

"Nick? Who's Nick?"

"He's the other guy I'm seeing."

"You're seeing three guys?"

"Yeah."

"Nick is single. That's good, right?"

"I guess. But I *love* Sam. I'd make such a great girlfriend."

It was not my business, really. As her sponsor it was my business to help her weigh and measure her food and refrain from sugar and flour. I once again invoked our food plan as a blueprint for living.

"You *love* Häagen-Dazs," I said.

"Dulce de leche," she said, her voice sultry with longing.

"But you can't have it. You can't have a scoop because you'll eat the whole pint and after that you'll eat everything you lay hands on. Are you with me?"

"Yeah . . ."

"OK. No Häagen-Dazs. But you have food you *can* eat, if you weigh and measure it. Even OK food is dangerous. Like your salad dressing. Maybe men are like that. You can't have some of men because you'll eat them up. Some men, like Nick, you *can* have, in a sane dose. Can you live with that today?"

"I might have to if things don't work out this afternoon. Sam's supposed to make a delivery in Brooklyn today. I hope so, anyway."

Like I said, most days she drove me batshit.

I could *not*, for one minute, understand how she lived in so much muddle. Couldn't she, I harrumphed, at *least* have started looking for a job before her benefits ran out? Terminate the affair? Wait until her divorce was final?

Listening to her made me grateful for my simple life. It also stirred my curiosity. *I'd make such a great girlfriend.*

What, I wondered as I grabbed my briefcase, *did that* mean?

Not much activity on the Intergalactic Men's Radio channel for me, I thought sourly on the train to work. I could count the incidents on one hand. Rick of the Warrens' deck the summer before had been the strongest signal. A nice guy, cute, and utterly unsuitable in every single way. Not worth regretting, and I never had.

Then there was my client and old friend, Ned. Two years earlier I had joined him at a writers' conference at Flathead in a dog-and-pony show for a flock of aspiring authors. I loved Ned, a talented memoirist of various macho pursuits, motorcycles and thirty-five years as a tree surgeon. He is also a man of great tenderness, as apt to be listening to a Beethoven quartet in his big truck as Marvin Gaye or the Doors.

It wasn't a serene prospect, mixing with Montana writers. I could have been one of them, had I stayed, had I kept writing. For the first time on that visit home, my new size 10 suit hanging in the closet, I wasn't thinking about my body.

I drove down to Yellow Bay to take Ned and his wife, Sarah, out for a drink at the conference cocktail hour. I didn't recognize anyone as I got directions to their cabin and, when I knocked and got no response, I began to think I could write a note and make a quick exit.

Ned appeared then, yawning and slightly disheveled from a nap. He gave me a squint-eyed look of suspicion, earned from the peculiar visitors he'd had since his book was published.

Not a glimmer of recognition.

"Oh, I woke you," I apologized. "I'm sor—"

"Frances? Oh my God—*Frances*?"

It wasn't a long beat of nonrecognition. As I'd found in Applebee's with my family, my voice was the tip-off. Later, over my seltzer and his gin, he grinned sheepishly. "You're probably sick of hearing this," he said, "but it's remarkable. You're beautiful." He laughed and slapped his hand on the picnic table. "How long have we known each other, anyway? Twenty years? I've never seen you blush!"

The next day Sarah told me she had returned with their two children from Glacier to an overcharged gossip mill. Writers, of course, are hopeless gossips, and this grows exponentially when they're locked up together with nothing to do but cabin-hop and worry about each other's successes. The scuttlebutt came back quickly. Ned was having an *affair*. While his wife was two hours away with their baby son and daughter! He'd been seen drinking with the woman—in plain sight. Ned Berensen had no shame.

Sarah told the informant that I was Ned's literary agent. An hour later the rumor had taken a new twist. Ned Berensen was sleeping with his agent.

We laughed at the absurdity of it. Ned's life is a paean to his love for Sarah. But the rumor wasn't sneering even if it wasn't true, and the incident came back to me once in a while as something more than an amusing variation on *All's Well That Ends Well*.

That was almost two years ago. Now it was really and truly spring in Brooklyn. Roses bloomed against the buildings as tulips collapsed into failed husks. People peeled off more clothes every day. I bounced into Eamon's to meet Dennis and his friend, Grace, in high spirits. Grace was visiting from Milan, as close to a civilian girlfriend as I had and a clotheshorse of the finest order. I would admire her latest moon boots and we'd talk frocks and my latest eBay jewelry. Dennis would be in good form for the occasion of her visit and a night spent with his two best friends.

A man put his hand on the bar stool next to me and asked if it was taken.

"It will be," I answered.

"But is it now?"

"No," I said, studying the obviousness of its emptiness. There were other stools available; it would be no problem to regroup when Dennis and Grace arrived, but my snottiness carried the day. He walked away.

Minutes later it occurred to me that the other seats were available for him as well as for us. I cycled through the three sentences we'd exchanged. Was it the location at the end of the bar, across from the patio that he'd wanted? I'd been up before five every morning that week, I was wan and there were circles under my eyes; I'd been reading in bed and my hair had gone

Flying Nun; I was feeling exposed and fat in my jeans and Mr. Rogers sweater. I hadn't really looked at him, but he had to be ten years younger than I. I was smoking and drinking coffee, abstractedly watching baseball on the TV over the bar—there was no come-hither in my posture. Was it the TV he wanted a view of?

When Grace and Dennis arrived, I waited impatiently through the double-kiss greetings and the arrangements of scooping themselves onto stools. My knee was jiggling as I told them about it. "Was that—you know—a—you know—?"

"A pickup?" Dennis finished for me. "No. But it might have been the beginning of a conversation, Frances." He squinched his eyes, calculating. "The pickup would've come with the fourth glass of wine." He turned to Grace. "Wouldn't you say?"

"Oh, God, Dennis, I don't know. It's been so long since anyone tried to pick me up. Get used to it, Frances."

"I guess I have to figure out when 'it's' happening, don't I?"

"So go out on a date," Grace said, and reached for the potato chips. "I'm eating like a pig, you know? I come to the States and I eat out and get all the food I can't get in Italy. I'm fat as a pig. I don't know how you do it."

I grimaced, still thinking about that kid, that man, regretting my pig-headed habit of general hostility. A date? I didn't know how to do anything.

My first date was an old work buddy Chris's fault. She had taken a new job as a senior editor and we met at a Rockefeller Center trattoria to celebrate our new employments. We had tales to tell, of what prompted us to leave our old jobs and the mandates and expectations of the new ones, and it was an easy setting for business talk, pretty but not painfully formal, among

other businesspeople schmoozing among the banquettes, the
tourists detoured by the promise of the sign outside, "Wine
Bar," that would make them too sleepy to hit FAO Schwarz,
Tiffany's, and MOMA before five o'clock. Chris munched her
salade niçoise and told me about an Internet dating guide she
had wanted to buy.

"Oof," I said. "Dating. I need to take lessons."

"You should try Match-dot-com. Men your age, they're different."

"No kidding," I answered dryly, picturing the debris and
fallout of divorced men trying to pass for human.

"No, not weird. Different from how they were ten or twenty
years ago. They've learned from their experiences, thought
about things. They're aware. And the demographics are on your
side."

I had to take her seriously—she sees every dating and relationship proposal that comes down the pike. I wrote it down.
"Match.com." In case, God help me, the time ever came.

And then it did.

Maybe it was Pam's successes with men, although I wouldn't
have called them that. Tearfully, she had consigned, at his insistence, New Jersey Sam to the status of dulce de leche and fret-
fully went on with the available guy she didn't love. She had
other dates as well, scouting the Planet of Men for arable land.

"It was such a nice afternoon," she said of a date at the
South Street Seaport. "We ate and walked around. He talked, I
laughed. He put me in a cab and kissed me goodbye and hasn't
called since. I don't get it. We had a good time." It was six days
after her date and we were standing on Montague Street watching the couples. Couples with toddlers. Teenaged lovers showing off their latest piercings. Couples at brunch with other
couples, or sleepily and secretly alone with each other. Couples
with dogs. With in-laws, informing them, "This is Brooklyn
Heights. We call it the Heights." With maps in Norwegian and
German and Japanese. With growing kids gulping up the

chance to tell Mom and Dad everything about their weeks. How had they all gotten from the awkward first date to lives that couldn't be separated?

"It's too bad for him," Pam went on with a toss of her blond hair and a clunk of her mahjong-tile earrings. "I'd have made him a wonderful girlfriend."

I agreed, but what did I know? What did it take to be a girlfriend? The mating rituals passing by flung me back to the Planet of Fat. What did they have that I didn't? I hadn't had a date yet and I was already confronted with the problem of whether I was girlfriend material. Whatever that was. Some ineffable quality contained in "The Girl I Marry," baby powder, and vanilla. *Pink*. I was definitely not pink.

So, I reasoned, I'm either not girlfriend material and should *(a)* enroll in arcane adult education classes for the next forty years, *(b)* give up and kill myself, or *(c)* actually meet one of these strange creatures—men—for a date.

Learning Latin could wait, and so could opening a vein. I'd know soon enough.

I took forty-eight hours to tiptoe around Match.com and consign my MasterCard to them. *Why not,* I figured. *It's just pen pals, no one has to know what planet I'm from.* It would be good to write to a real live heterosexual man.

It was harder than I thought. "What body type am I?" I begged of Bridget and Amy. I was losing weight again, slowly; Bridget had another twenty pounds for me to go. That put me in Match-dot's "a few extra pounds" category, right? "No," they said firmly, in unison. The other choices were "slim/slender" and "normal." "You're *normal,* Frances," Bridget insisted. "You have a normal body."

"Describe yourself," it asked. "I am sick of books," I wrote, "hungry to DO things, live a little vividly." I refused ownership of myself, paraphrasing what friends said about my looks and qualities. Noting that I looked at profiles of men with photos, I found one I could countenance, taken at a giggly Saturday lunch with Tracy. It caught me laughing, my eyes scrunched in conspiratorial merriness. I liked that picture a lot.

By the time my photograph was posted, I was in the beginnings of an email correspondence with a man in another city, a photographer. "Great smile," he wrote.

I sat back in my chair, hard. *Information.* It had come from a handsome man who knows about women's faces.

"Have you ever," he asked in an early email, "walked barefoot on the beach at dawn, holding hands, saying nothing?"

Sharp breath, then cynicism kicked in. Had he been hanging out in the Hallmark poster section? Was this a come-on? I didn't know and I didn't care. I cast my lot with that first cold stab of breath. Which turned quickly into denouncement. *No, damn it, I haven't. I've been shut* out! *I've been denied!!*

Then I remembered. Fifteen years ago, I'd sat on the porch of a hillside restaurant in Missoula, drinking gin and tonics with the man I'd been hopelessly in love with since we were twenty-one. The northeastern horizon plumped against the stars, glowed, pulsed, faded. "The Northern Lights," I whispered, as though my voice would crack the apparition.

"Amazing," he agreed, and turned to me. "I'm buying you a huckleberry milkshake tomorrow. 'Cause you saw 'em first."

I wanted to do a Bette Davis about my tragically solo life— "It's *Aunt* Vale; every family has one, you know"—but in such irregular moments, I'd had minutes of perfect accord and union. I had shared, with Chris of the Northern Lights, nights of swimming naked in Flathead Lake, the moon wallowing like a pancake in molasses. There was a sunset we'd chased as we yammered excitedly about *A Fish Named Wanda*. He had woken me up once, wonderfully, at four in the morning, tipsy on Christmas eggnog, with nothing to say but wanting to hear my voice. If his idea of our romance was, when I confessed my feelings for him, that we should get married, but to other people and tell each other about our marriages, I had to admit those swims and those synchronous enthusiasms *had* taken place. It was still romantic.

My friends, too, had been the companions of my heart. My first San Gennaro Festival with Richard, a pal from graduate school, drinking red wine with peach slices and laughing at the oom-pah band straight out of *The Godfather* was another synchronicity. Platonic, yes, but still romantic. I pictured Dennis standing under the portico at Lincoln Center, looking like Gary Cooper in his leather trench coat, seen through a graph of rain. Romance was being eighteen years old and sleeping in a parking lot at Lake McDonald with Kim, waking to a dawn so cold the lake was steaming, Cat Stevens the soundtrack.

Take it one step further, and when wasn't I in love? I risked it every time I opened a new manuscript. I had shelves of lives I'd been seduced by.

I knew how to give my heart away.

I had been romantic if not romanced.

Maybe—just—I knew more than I thought I knew.

Dennis was appalled and fascinated by online dating.

"It seems so—*bald*." He cocked his head and pondered the smoke curling lazily from his cigarette in the June humidity. We were sitting on Montague Street, boy-watching and boy-talking.

"Why?" I asked.

"I don't know. I think you should meet men naturally."

I snorted. Dennis's method of finding men involved occasionally answering a personal in the *New York Review of Books,* and a lot of drinking in the swankier gay bars that resulted in frequently being stood up for dinner dates the next night.

"*I* don't drink," I said snappishly. "*I'm* too old for singles bars, whatever they are. Maybe gay men can keep doing it into decrepitude, but it kind of loses interest for straight women. Who would I meet? Some drunk guy? No, thanks."

Still, his interest was piqued. We went home and I fired up the website. "Cool!" he said as pictures popped up of the few men who met his requirements of age, smoking, drinking, and locality—he was ready to let education and income go. Then he turned brutally to business, stripping them of any redeeming qualities, but impressed by the technology and the numbers that I, as a straight woman, had at my fingertips.

"You *know* how much I love catalogue shopping," I said.

I preferred initiating contact. Being trolled caught me off guard, and made me defensive. My regular Match-dot correspondent was a three-hour train trip away. I was ready to make the trip, or take a day off from work to meet him, but this, that, and another thing always bollixed his calendar. Skilled at unrequited love, I began to agonize.

"Fran," Dr. Miller reasoned, "this is ambivalence. He sort of wants someone so he puts himself up there but he's not following through. It's *three hours.* Tell him you're coming down, you'll be at the station at noon, and you'll have lunch. Even if he doesn't show up, you'll have a nice day."

Inform him—tell him—expect? Not fucking likely, I beetle-browed back at her. Didn't she know how lucky I was that such a dishy guy was writing and calling me?

I'd sort of gotten the First Law About Men on the Warrens' dock last summer when I realized that if a man asks if you're single and available, he's interested. It took Mr. Match.com's inertia to teach me the Second Law: they're either *There,* ready for the moment and the possibilities, or they aren't.

We emailed each other at least once a day, notes about our lives. How his cats reacted to a flea bath (unhappily), how my first attempt at cold poached salmon turned out (very well), the headshots he took of an actress (they would have been better if she'd worn makeup), our songs du jour (Annie Lennox's "Downtown Lights" in New York, Moby's "Porcelain" three hours south). Once a week or so he called, sometimes on his cell phone because he'd run late and didn't want me to wait up till he got home. We told our stories and compared notes on the gym and movies and neighbors. These were long conversations, without endearments but convivial and mutual. "We should meet," I would gather my courage to say every third or fourth phone call, and he agreed.

So it wasn't that he didn't like me. He did. But the Third Law About Men is that they don't know if they're *There* or not. They think they are. They will pay money to list themselves at Match-dot or the Right Stuff or in the back of *New York Magazine,* but it's a twinge of loneliness that fools them into thinking they are ready for the possibilities of a companion. Like a headache, it passes but you keep aspirin on hand. Just in case.

If he'd asked, I'd have jumped on Amtrak and been there for coffee.

But he acted under the assumption that there was time. Maybe, in time, he'd be *There,* which, to him, was almost the same as being *There,* which meant he might as well put up his profile on Match-dot.

Which leaves the judging of There/Not There up to women. Up, in short, to *me.*

. . .

He was the right man for that season. I needed to go slow, but
as the summer ground into New York nonmotion I began to
suspect that emailing was not dating.

I needed to know if I could look a man in the eye and still
find things to talk about. More important, I shuddered, could
he look *me* in the eye and want to keep looking? What would
men *see*, how would my body rate? Was I pretty enough? Was
I soft-tempered and easy to talk to? What kind of package
was I?

Was I . . . pink?

Then a Match-dot found me. I gave him my phone number and
I liked his gentle voice, although I was irked when he told me
he liked my profile because he thought I could give him a reading list.

I agreed to meet him for coffee late Sunday afternoon—my
first date in nine years, the second date in my life.

What will Vanna wear tonight? I asked my closet as I spun
the wheel of fortune for a five o'clock coffee date in August.
Clothes were scattered at my feet. Too serious, too formal, too
big, today it feels too small. Too black.

Über-Frances stepped in with lists. *What do you want to say?*
she asked Scaredy-cat Frances, agog at the hangers of shirts.
Make a list.

Maybe. I want to say maybe.

Camisole.

But I can't show my arms.

Sweater.

No pressure. I want to say no pressure.

Loose trousers.

Girlie. Summery.

Linen. Cream colored. Hurry. You have ten minutes to get to Montague Street.

My date was wearing jeans split at the knees and a faded T-shirt, and he carried a Peruvian satchel very much like one I had in college. I wasn't surprised when he described his yoga class and involvement in liberal Brooklyn causes.

"So," he shifted from himself to me, "what happened?"

I crossed my arms protectively over my chest, tugging my sweater together. "What do you mean?"

"You've never been married. What's the story?"

"No story," I said breezily. "I forgot."

"You forgot to get married?"

I sighed. This was the hard part. "I lost 175 pounds. I finished two years ago. I've been morbidly obese my entire life and I—"

"A hundred and seventy-five pounds?" He whistled softly.

"I didn't want to start dating until I was reasonably certain I could keep it off."

That was one of the heavy pieces of baggage attached to my story. I was also telling him, if he was smart and could read between the lines, that I do not have a pretty body. The residual damage is extensive, and Dr. Miller's reassurances that every middle-aged body carries its share of aging did not comfort me. A man who was interested in me should be prepared for what was under the Liz Claiborne.

"How does it feel? It must be amazing to be so much lighter."

"It's not like I took a 170-pound backpack off," I said for the millionth time. "It wasn't one big weight in one place. I lost weight in my fingers and feet. Places you never think about."

"Still," he insisted, "it must make a huge difference."

"I run incredibly cold," I offered.

"I was wondering why you're wearing a sweater."

"So," I tossed the ball back in his court, "what's your story? You haven't been married, either, right?"

But he had the saving caveat for never-married people in their forties, a "long-term live-in relationship." "She was crazy," he explained. Six months after the relationship had ended, he decided to join Match-dot.

And here we were.

We had dinner and went on to haltingly introduce the rest of our lives. He was a textbook editor and worked at home. To his overeager questions about being a literary agent, I gave easy answers, cautious about whether he would start telling me about a novel he was finishing. This was not smugness. I'd actually had a Match-dot email me his short stories to evaluate. To his questions about my opinion of Joyce and Beckett, I laughed. "I gave up having to talk about them when I dropped out of graduate school." He was disappointed at having his fantasy of a lit chick popped. I felt bad about that—wasn't part of girlfriend material being interesting and interested? At that moment, I couldn't care less for literature. I was on an odyssey for true romance.

He offered to walk me to the bank as I writhed about how we would say goodbye. My discomfort was dispelled when I caught the eye of a dog in front of Starbucks. There is nothing I love more than a dog desperately in need of having its ears scratched, the cardinal rule being that every dog needs its ears scratched. It flopped on its back as I doggie-talked to its grinning pleasure. "Wooza-wooza-wooza, voo wants a belly-rub, don't voo?" Its tail could have whipped cream as it sneezed in excitement. Ears, belly, a twist to its feet for a butt-rub to finish the job, and I was ready to move on. My date, however, was stopped in his tracks.

"How'd you *do* that?"

"What?"

"That dog. He . . . like, he melted for you."

"Babies and dogs," I answered. "What can I say? They love me."

Later that night, I got an email thanking me for a nice evening, but after further reflection he had decided he wasn't "over" his last relationship. I was not, apparently, able to inspire him to move on, but then it ain't over 'til the fat lady sings, a thought that gave me enough mirth to make up for failure. Maybe it wasn't *our* first date, but it was *mine*. I was in shopping rather than buying mode, and I'd given the merchandise a look.

Score one for the Girl.

I came to think of my summer of dating as applying for immigration and naturalization. I'd gotten to Earth and was passing for human; now I was considering the options of what nation would accept my application for a green card.

I began referring to my dates as countries. My out-of-towner, my favorite, was New Zealand. His idiosyncrasies were like the counterclockwise draining of water south of the Equator. A musician who emailed me from the studio at 3 A.M. for two months became Transylvania. The first date, with his leftist local politics and yoga classes, was Sweden. Liberal, humanitarian, dull.

There were a number of Swedish knock-offs. I was consciously contacting men who were . . . well . . . ugly. My reasoning was that if he didn't look like a movie star, surely he would forgive my own physical flaws. Always, always the forgiveness was for my wrinkled sagging venous scarred body.

They were mostly nice men, the Swedes, but they were moles,

with strange jobs, or no jobs, that allowed too much time at home. They made me grateful I had to leave the house in business clothes, that my "free" time was full of manuscripts, the Stepfords, Dr. Miller, the gym, chores. I was not a mole.

I wanted them to wear their second-best pair of jeans. I wanted them to own more than one pair of jeans.

I amassed passport stamps from Holland, Israel, and Canada. Holland was a lawyer who had written "love dancing at midnight" in his profile but turned out to be on disability leave. Israel had definite ideas about how to make moussaka, why I should not listen to Benny Goodman, and how learning to golf would save my soul. He could even do a better job of teaching me in the weight room than my physical trainer. Israel, I told Dennis, was better than Super Cable.

Canada pushed me over the edge and it was my own fault. After two months, I wanted to be kissed, wanted to have sex. I wanted proof that I was a Girl. I didn't care, by Labor Day, what he did or looked like. We met at a coffee shop near Columbia and I soon learned he was the king of the amateurs. He did not work, subsisting instead on renting half of his apartment to a graduate student in order to organize the beautification of his Upper West Side neighborhood and play the piano. "I'm kind of proud of having no visible means of support," he told me as we sat in the sun. He'd chosen this coffee shop for the bottomless refill he graciously offered to buy. "It's made me spiritual. *You* should try it."

"Really?" I said, shaking my head when he offered me one of his cigarettes and lighting one of my own. "Why?"

"For instance, twice a year I fast for a month. I don't have anything except water, coffee, and fruit juice. It saves money, gives me discipline, *and* keeps me thin. It's interesting," he segued, "how all the women I've met from Match-dot say they're thin or average, when they should be in the next category. Like you. You are clearly 'a few extra pounds.' "

My spine stiffened and I dropped my cigarette to the pavement. I ground it hard. I wished it was him.

"I hope you don't mind me saying that."

"I didn't pick the category lightly and I didn't pick it alone." I stopped. I didn't want to bore him with facts—that the average size of American women is 14 and I was a 10, that I carried maybe fifteen pounds of skin I could do nothing about, that compared to what I once was . . . I could go on and on but, despite the lump in my throat, I was determined to try to make a go of this date.

So I stopped. And I accepted his invitation to see his shared apartment and the computer he'd assembled from parts he found on the street. We kissed and immediately he slid my dress up my ass.

"Can we go a little slower?" I asked, sliding his hand and my dress down.

"Of course," he said, and hugged me tight.

And kept hugging.

I was not there for hugging. I turned my face and kissed the side of his mouth, inviting more. He pressed me hard again, cheek to cheek, and rocked me. "Hugging is nice," he said.

"Yeah," I answered cautiously. "I have a zillion friends I *hug.*" I kissed the side of his mouth again, a little harder.

"Actually." He let me go. "It's your breath."

I had two physical movements I was capable of in that flash. My jaw closed hard; my hand slapped a manhole cover over my mouth. *Shit. I knew I shouldn't have smoked on a date.*

Wait. He smokes—those vile black cigarettes from Romania. He probably finds them in some Slavic history professor's trash.

I stepped back. "May I use your toothpaste?"

He had a bleak apologetic expression to hand me. "That's not it. It's something you eat, something gastric. Maybe you need to fast for a month and subsequently eat only brown rice."

That's when I started crying.

What was I thinking, I excoriated myself on the train home. *He owns one pair of jeans.* He had bragged about finding them in a Columbia dorm Dumpster.

I was sobbing when I got back to Brooklyn and ran into a Stepford named Jennifer. Stepfords are like that. They materialize out of thin air when I need them most.

Jennifer was exactly who I needed. I'd watched her with a certain fascinated alarm in the Rooms, afraid of her moxie but tantalized by the way she moved through life as though she cast no shadow. She was brazen in everything she did, including bringing her pony-sized dog to the Rooms without asking whether pets were allowed, and walking around in tatters when it was 50 degrees outside.

Jennifer wore sunglasses at night.

I was startled when I overheard her talking about a boyfriend. I'd assumed she was a biker dyke and that someday she would order me up in front of the Lesbian Tribunal for Failure to Be Gay.

"Hey!" she called as I walked out of the Clark Street station. "Frances!" I looked up as she glided over to me. "What's up, babe?"

More tears trickled down my nose at "babe." I didn't know this woman except in careful passing, but "babe" brought out the baby in me.

"I had a date. He . . . he didn't like me, I guess. I wanted him to. I tried, but"—I hiccupped a sob—"it didn't work."

"No, honey, no," she shouted at me. "You're doin' it all wrong, Miss Thing. You gotta come up to my roof while I explain a few things to you."

She was accompanied by her dog, Godiva, and Jake, a hyper white Lab. How could I say no?

Jennifer alternately cajoled and idolized Jake as he raced up and down the rooftop thirty-five floors above the skyline of Wall Street. He dashed off to a sunbather and buried his snout in her crotch, making my tutorial with Jennifer staccato and a little hard to follow. Finally she snapped his leash on and bribed him with Liv-A-Snaps to lie down.

"Jesus, he's a maniac. Aren't you, baby? He's spoiled rotten at home—look how fat he is. He's only ten months old, for God's sake." Jennifer was a former Trundler. She had a prosperous dog-walking business, an alternative she preferred to her former life as a lawyer. One hundred and seventy pounds heavier, she couldn't have done this job. Through her work, she was, de facto, the mayor of Montague Street, well acquainted with the 2,256 dogs in Brooklyn Heights and, by association, their owners. The owners took their lives in their hands if they didn't shoot square with Jennifer. By the time we got to her rooftop I knew she was the least bullshitting woman I'd ever meet. Of the dogs, however, she adored 98.5 percent of them; their opinion of her ran 100 percent paws-up. I trusted the dogs and therefore trusted her.

"OK, Frances, get a grip," she said with no pity in her voice. "First of all, this guy is a loser, OK? If he wasn't blown away by you it's only proof of how stupid he is."

"Yeah, but he said I'd lied about my weight on Match-dot. That I should have said 'a few extra pounds.' " I looked down at my butter-yellow linen dress. It was way too big but living in the Fun House Mirror was bewildering. Was it the dress? My vanity? His demented expectations? My body?

"You look *fab*ulous, darling. You know that, don't you?" She peered at me over the rim of her dark glasses, her eyes hard as obsidian. "Don't. You."

I swallowed and nodded.

"You don't have much experience but trust me, you scare the hell out of these guys. Use it. I've been with a lot of men. A *lot*. And they're all jerks. You have nothing to prove. They have to prove themselves to *you,* got it? Stop going out with moles. Go for looks, see what happens. Maybe nothing, but it won't be any worse than walking away from a mole man, believe me. I know. Don't I, Jakey?" Whap, whap went his Labrador tail, hard as a sock full of marbles. Fast as falling table scraps, Jake was on his feet and tangled in his leash with the certainty that food was to be had. He jumped into my lap and I buried my hands and face in the fur and loose skin at his neck. His head reared up to get a good close look at me before he started licking my face with wild avidity.

At least Jake didn't mind my breath.

"I'm doing it one more time," I told Pam when she asked whether she should have coffee with the married man's best (and single) friend. "We gotta try, and we gotta know when to stop. I'll contact the three cutest guys I might be able to talk to. After that I give up."

13

CITIZENSHIP

I t was now or never. I wasn't fooling around.
My requirements were not numerous.

Besides owning two pairs of jeans, Mystery Date must
- not ask me to read his novel, short stories, or poetry;
- make me laugh and laugh at my jokes;
- leave the house with a specific destination at least three
  times a week to earn a living;
- not tell me how to cook, what to read, what music to
  listen to, what to do at the gym;
- let me do what I have to do without hoo-haw—no

comments on my big salads, seeing the Stepfords, getting up at five in the morning on weekends, obsession
with clothes;

• notice the day—the smell of coffee and how sunlight
  gets tangled in the trees.

This was reasonable, surely. We could refine as we went
along. It would be nice, for instance, if he knew the difference
between a metaphor and a simile and found my salt-and-pepper
shaker collection endearing. I'd swoon if he had been known to
weep over Mahler's Symphony no. 4, but I was wise enough to
know that where swooning is involved, lecturing and proscrib-
ing were waiting in the wings.

For my part, I was ready to *offer* to read his novel, listen and
applaud, make time in my schedule, make soup, and clean the
bathroom.

That was fair, surely.

Good conversations came out of the last three Match-dots.
I'd become adept at assigning them nationalities. The first man I
talked to was a Frenchman, with obscure literary references and
a profile that claimed suaveness; the second was a Spaniard, full
of heated poetry and maleness; there was a chatty email from a
man bob-bob-bobbing along in Connecticut, describing a morning in a used bookstore and an evening with a friend's new computer. Canadian blandness? Swiss neutrality? Whatever. I had
men to meet the week after Labor Day. I'd even nailed the Transylvanian to a lunch date.

On September 10, 2001, after long conversations and lots of
flirtation, the Spaniard decided to pick me up from work and
take me to dinner. He arrived in an SUV with two Winnebago-
sized dogs in back, Bouviers—Booves—bigger than Jennifer's
dog by far. The late-night conversations of the weekend dis-
solved in the drenching rain we navigated to Brooklyn and in
the negotiation of finding a restaurant with dry outdoor tables
so the Booves could join us for dinner. He drank a Coke and de-

scribed Krakowesque adventures, Indiana Jones meets George Smiley. I listened and said encouraging things and wished he had more hair. Still, he wasn't trying to tell me how to cook eggplant or which Wilkie Collins novel I should read next. *Maybe,* I thought as I ate my broccoli rabe in too much oil. *Maybe with time.* Maybe he'd be a great lover. If only he'd ask me one question about myself or shut up for one second.

The best part of the evening was seeing Jennifer a half block away coming back from a late dog-walking gig, her own Bouvier, Godiva, in stately and complacent tow. "Jennifer," I yelled, and shot out of my chair to run down to Henry Street. "I have a surprise for Godiva. Come on." We convened the shaggy blue-gray ponies disguised as dogs as Señor pontificated on the breed and Jennifer's presence collected yet more dogs and their owners. Godiva was nonplussed at the story of her Belgian origins and distinctly nonplussed by the new bitches on the block although she had some momentary activity around a dapper boxer before she lay down on the sidewalk and fell asleep at Jennifer's feet.

The Spaniard kissed me chastely good night and promised to call—maybe we'd take the dogs to the beach that weekend. I went home thinking smutty thoughts in which he miraculously grew more hair.

"Hello, darling," Jennifer growled into the phone an hour later. "How *are* you?"

"Do you like him?"

"Darling, he is a class A asshole. I've never seen more obese Booves, and I've been with a lot of Bouviers. A *lot.*"

"So?" I asked. "The dogs are overweight, so what?

"Love means never letting your dog go to the dogs. You do that, you'll let your girlfriend go to the dogs, too. Only in your case, you should go to the dogs. Or get a dog. At least they let you do some of the talking. I love you. Good night." She hung up, leaving me to ignore her dislike.

I was daydreaming about him as I worried how late I was for

work the next morning. The train pulled into Cortlandt Street and the mass exit of worker bees crowded out while the train waited. I looked at my watch—it was a little after nine—and went back to thinking about what I'd wear to the beach that weekend. The train waited. I heard a boom; the train rocked a little. People looked up incuriously and shook their papers back into place. Then the conductor announced that we were to exit the train and leave the station.

As we breached the street, I turned and hissed at the woman pushing me, "Calm down. We're almost out—everything's fine."

It was not fine. It was ticker tape noodling the air of a periwinkle day. A car on the sidewalk with its windows smashed. A man standing at the head of the stairs, leaning against a Learning Annex box, looking raptly up. He was so riveted that my gaze crawled along his, a hundred floors up to the World Trade Center, which had a bite taken out of it and was on fire.

On September 11, I was able to run. I ran from the tsunami of people speed-marching out of the Towers, I ran from the bodies like slowly spinning propellers falling from the melting sky, I ran from the shrieking parade of emergency vehicles that would not, could not, stop for pedestrians.

My weight loss had saved my life.

Startled by sudden noises, riddled with sirens, New Yorkers became almost tender in their protection of each other for a few weeks. The Frenchman called that night to make sure I was OK, as did my New Zealander three hours south. The Señor went into manly action to save lives. His obese Booves, it turned out, were trained to sniff out bodies.

"Yeah," Jennifer drawled. "And then probably *eat* them.

Don't waste your time wondering why he doesn't call, honey. Move on."

I did. I had lunch with my Transylvanian, not as interesting as his enigmatic profile and picture on Match-dot, and frankly insulting when he complained about fat people. "You know," he went on, half accusingly. "How they take up so much *space*? You can't get around them and they walk so *slow*. Do they do that on purpose?"

"I'm really not allowed to address that," I answered coldly. "The Federation of Fat People obligates us not to tell its secrets after we've taken a leave of absence."

Oh, well.

I met the Frenchman for drinks at a midtown hotel bar that always amused me. Done up in what could be Dalí's Eve of St. Agnes dream, it stirred Versailles, the Flintstones, and the first *Star Trek Enterprise* together in no particular order. I dressed up that day, not for him but because I refused to be ready to run. Nor could I, not in the shoes I'd chosen for my statement.

I took a seat—or a throne—next to a Plexiglas table and ordered a stiff seltzer, pulled out a sheaf of manuscript, and started reading. I badly wanted to smoke but smoking is such a make-or-break habit on first dates that I gritted my teeth and waited.

"Frances," Monsieur said. "I'm glad I recognized you."

I was too. He looked nothing like his picture on Match-dot.

He set his leather satchel down, nodded to the waitress, and asked for a Gray Goose on the rocks.

"Good thing, me recognizing you." He smiled sweetly. "My photo, I must admit, was taken forty pounds ago."

"Oh," I said, flustered. What was I supposed to say? I'd heard stories like this, they're rife in the online and personals dating world. It occurred to me that this was payback for Mr. Canada. "It was a great photo," I offered. "That's why I emailed you."

"Thanks. It's my favorite picture, that's why I use it."

No it's not, I thought as I smiled encouragingly. *He isn't ugly*, I told myself. *Lots of normal women are with bigger men. I see 'em all the time.*

"I can see why—you look so happy in it."

"It was taken in Woodstock. I go up there on buying expeditions. And I still have the smile."

And anyway, I went on, *he's a man.*

Men get away with forty pounds and women don't. Men get away with thinning and/or gray hair and women don't. I didn't think these gender laws were fair but I couldn't fight an entire culture.

Maybe he'll make me laugh. Maybe I'll make him laugh. I crossed my legs and admired my white-stockinged kneecaps under layers of navy blue chiffon, waggled my ankle. I was in no position to point my finger at a man's physical flaws. I was only passing for thin, after all, with lots of hair coloring and hot wax supplementing my looks. It would be a hard call to determine the greater liar between us.

He was a genuinely nice man, an importer of luxury items from Europe, a wine and restaurant lover. But then there was the "but" factor. He didn't make me laugh, I didn't feel like he had anything new to inspire me to learn. In the end, the goofiness of the bar's décor that matched the Cosmopolitans the few posttrauma customers dawdled over was more compelling.

The emails from Connecticut were sorrowful and concerned, as yet without a nationality. He wrote of his bafflement and sense of futility after Tuesday's events, with no other opinion attached. By the time the wind shifted on the morning of the twelfth, carrying bits of office documents and smoke off to New Jersey, I was having the same nonreaction to it. I wrote that people were having lunch on the sidewalk cafés, and Key Food was selling hazelnut coffee as usual. The city was closed on the twelfth and people were taking the day off in the usual New York fashion. Lunch, the Gap, a latte, and a stroll down to the Promenade to watch the plumes of smoke, then home to more loops of the same footage we'd been watching for thirty hours. I thought this was just fine, I wrote him. New York wasn't stopping its rituals for anything. It made me proud.

We exchanged stories of how each of us had bottomed out and landed in church basements reciting the twelve steps, although for different addictions. He sent me a picture of his son, massively overweight and begging the camera with the sad eyes and defeated smile I recognized from my own seventh-grade pictures. I emailed back that there were two things he needed to do: tell anyone who asked the boy whether he'd like to lose weight to shut the fuck up, and tell the boy it was not his fault.

The emails from Connecticut turned into real flirtations. Dennis and I had recently had a long discussion on the anatomy of kissing, and kissing was on my mind. I wanted to date a really first-rate kisser. "What do you think of kissing?" I wrote him, and his answer was worthy of Emily Dickinson: "Oh, oh! snowflakes, piling up, light, dancing."

I had to get up from my computer and take a walk after reading that.

I emailed him my phone number.

He called on a Monday night when I was into a four-Sominex sleep.

His voice made me think of butterscotch, the taste and the color. Mellow and even and light.

"I woke you, didn't I?"

"Yes," I said groggily, pulling myself up in bed and reaching for the lamp. "But it's fine. I love being woken up by a man."

It was the truth. Was it my fault it could be construed as provocative?

He laughed a little awkwardly. "I'm sorry. I could call you tomorrow."

"No, no." I thumped my pillows into shape and pulled my knees up to my chin. "I'm awake now. How was your day, Ward?"

His laugh was genuine now, merry as Santa's elves waking up to Easter baskets. "Fine, June. What's for dinner?"

"Meat loaf, your favorite. We'll sit down as soon as Wally comes in from baseball."

"Did the Beav pass his math test?"

"Sadly, no. I've had to lock him in the attic with Gidget, Kitten, Princess, and . . ." My lexicon of television adolescents was running out.

"The Professor and Mary Ann?"

"That's right. Oh, Ward. You're such a good father."

"I am, you know," he said, taking a step beyond silly. "Tonight, for instance, we had Boy Scouts."

"Oh my."

"Yes. Scouts. Where they make men out of boys so they can make Republicans out of men."

"Really. Is there a badge for becoming a Republican, or is that after Eagle Scouts?"

"Neither, after tonight."

"Did you stage a coup?"

"Far from it. I was having a reasonable conversation with the Scout master after the meeting. He wants me to talk to the troop about computers or whatever. We're in the parking lot and we're talking and all of a sudden there's this beeping. Both of us grab our cell phones, but that's not it. It's this sort of shrill beeping. Then I remember. My Power Girls watch. I never have figured out how to set my Power Girls watch. I laugh and I hold out my wrist and I say, 'I never have figured out how to set my Power Girls watch,' and the Scout master starts sort of backing up—*skitch, skitch*. And I say, 'Supposedly it can do all kinds of things. Remind you when to save the world, and what boys to watch out for. But I lost the directions. Still . . .' He's almost to his car now, an SUV of course—"

"With a gun rack?" I interjected.

"Of course. So I say, 'It's a cool watch, don't you think?' "

"The poor man," I moaned, shaking my head against the

quilt tent over my knees. "You scared him to death. He probably thinks you want to date him."

"Good," he said. There was a harder note in that golden voice. "Maybe we'll get kicked out of Boy Scouts for homosexuality. The Power Girls would have done their job."

I emailed him an apology for how dopey I'd been that night, placing the blame on Sominex and a book deal I was negotiating at the office. "I can be funny, too," I claimed, and I was, a few nights later when I described a party for agents and how Alix had gotten us kicked out of the cabaret portion of the evening by getting drunk and insisting on hip-bumping in time to the music while complaining loudly about the singer. "So I say to her husband, 'You're a shrink, what's all this hip-bumping about?' 'Freud would say it's a latent masturbation fantasy,' he answers and I say, 'Well, *you're* the husband. Do something about it!' "

"OK, OK," he gasped. "I just had to lie down on the kitchen floor. What did you do next?"

"I thought about meeting you tomorrow. Under the big clock at Grand Central. I wondered what to wear."

"I've never even *talked* to someone this soon after email, let alone *met* them."

" 'This soon'? I've talked, met, and been sent home in shame in less time than one of our phone calls," I sputtered. "Are we going to meet?"

"I think we have to," he said. "I think your eyes are going to ask things. They'll want to go dancing, won't they?"

These were seductions, a cross between Petrarch and Mother Goose, with sound effects. And intuition running like a current of tornado-lightning through my bones.

. . .

Saturday was hot and tense with rumors of another terrorist strike in the city. Terror had already struck me. I liked him. What would come next? How did I let it, how did I encourage it to happen?

He was at the information desk in Grand Central, the tall blond he'd described himself to be. He was carrying a rose.

For me.

My eyes fell on it with dread. He faltered. "I brought this for you."

"Oh."

And so, filled with diffidence and making jokes about 1-800-Bad-Date ("We'll pick him up for $19.95 and deliver him to the train terminal of your choice!"), I cast about for what to do with the afternoon. My joking petered out and he began to talk. And talk and talk, as we had coffee and he showed me pictures of his son and I relaxed.

"Do you like kids?"

"I am a professional aunt. I'd actually prefer to meet someone with kids, if they play Monopoly. My nieces and nephews are out of the Monopoly circuit. I'm looking for replacements. Or victims."

He talked as we walked through sidewalk photo galleries of people missing from the World Trade Center, through the spontaneous Union Square shrine smelling of candle wax and incense, where he threaded the rose into a steel mesh fence. On down Broadway to Mulberry Street, where he put his hand on my shoulder as we crossed streets. *Is that . . . does that mean . . . ?* We ate lunch and I discovered he lived almost entirely on salads and he said I looked like a schoolmarm with a wicked streak when I put on my reading glasses. I gaped, thanked him, and a minute or two later undid the top button of my jacket. We kept heading south after lunch, through Chinatown. On Mott Street I turned to him as he continued to talk (about his son, about his childhood, about his coworkers, about Calvin and Hobbes) and nearly blurted, "Would you just *kiss* me?!" My face twitched, so on the brink I was—*say it, don't you* dare—that he paused in his chatter. I opened my mouth. I shut it. I opened it again, gawping like a hungry dolphin. I shook my head in anger at myself and walked across the street, leaving him to his own gawping.

An hour later we sat down on the fountain across from City Hall. He was telling me a story about a college friend and I was trying to think of what to do next. He'd professed indifference to seeing a movie, we'd already eaten, neither of us drank. That left—what? bowling? A carriage ride in Central Park? We were in New York City and I couldn't think of anything to do? *You are such an asshole, Frances,* I slapped myself. My brows darkened.

"I know you're fragile," he said, cutting off the story of going to a bar in Provincetown with his friend. He leaned over and kissed me on the cheek. *Oh great,* I thought. *He has cheek-kissing feelings for me. Next he'll tell me I remind him of the sister he always wanted.* "And I know you're scared and not very experienced." *And I don't want to be the one to hurt you,* I supplied for him. "But I'd really like to kiss you."

The italics stopped. I looked at him and said, nearly in tears, "For God's sake, I wish you would."

And he did. In the shadow of the missing World Trade Center towers, to the applause, eventually, of bystanders, until the fountain was turned off.

"What was the deal with the rose?" he asked the next day.

"I was embarrassed," I told him. "People would know we were on a *date*. I hate women with roses."

"As much as you hate people making out on subways?" he bubbled. "As much as you hate people like us?"

"I don't hate anyone more than people like us." I hugged his knee between mine. "At least it wasn't a balloon."

"No, dear," he answered. "A balloon would have been an *outing*."

"When did you know you were going to kiss me?"

"I wasn't at all sure when you met me at the station. You were so tense, I thought, uh-oh, this is a mistake. Then we had coffee and you smiled and that's when it happened. You have a smile that lights up a room."

He couldn't tell me that story often enough.

It was three lovely, revealing months: kissing on the campus of his Ivy League alma mater, being surprised and seduced by a single word, "Apoplectic," got me the first night; "gimcrack," referring to a shining expanse of Christmas ornaments in Saks could have gotten him any sexual favor he wanted. For three months we laughed and kissed and laughed.

Every turn of his mind amazed me. He answered idle questions so quickly, so deftly, that something inside me turned over. We would think of the same joke and say it simultaneously, our eyes dilating in astonishment. I was prepared to be utterly unprepared.

I was also prepared for his horrified reaction to my body. Luxuriating in bed one morning, I gasped when I realized I was lying without the quilt and yanked it to my chin. "Don't," he said. "I know what you had to do to get your body. It's beautiful."

Being told I was beautiful when we were making love was wonderful, but it earned its chops when I was in red flannel pajamas and my nerd bifocals, sitting on the floor wrapping Christmas presents. He turned from my computer to expound on the history of *Time* magazine's Man of the Year and laughed instead. "You're adorable right now."

He broke my weight loss down in ways I hadn't considered before. I had my arsenal of facts. Pounds, size, months. I knew what parts of my body I should flatter, and how to do it. With some cunning, and sometimes to his own surprise, he took pleasure in startling me with what my physical change added up to. "You can't do that!" I protested when he pulled me onto his lap or picked me up. I did not mean my space had been invaded, I meant he couldn't do it—no one could, no one ever had, I was not pick-upable. "Frances," he admonished, "you're *thin*. Don't you get it?"

"I'd hate to be the first man who told you that you're beautiful," he'd written before we met. Partly because he was, really, the first man to tell me that, I was confused by the statement. Did he know that such a compliment would make me snort in disbelief or dismissal, according to how much I liked the man? Did he fear how much convincing I'd need, and that of course I *wanted* to be convinced? Was he afraid of how draining the convincing would be for him? I didn't ask what he meant until much later and by then he'd formed his version of me.

Maybe he thought I was his son, grown up but needing excesses of love and attention, more than there was in the world. He described his son as a sucking black hole of need. Was there enough of him left after that?

Maybe he was right to be afraid. There was so much I needed to *know*.

"Honey," I half whispered, half whined as he was falling asleep the weekend of my birthday. "Why do you like me?" My birthday is complicated with feelings about being given away, not being what my parents hoped when they brought me home. I needed to know who and what I was.

He groaned. "Frances."

"Honey. Why?"

"Because you're beautiful and funny and I like your stuff. OK?"

The Good Doctor Miller groaned as well. "Fran. He was *in bed* with you. You have a *date* for New Year's Eve. What more do you want?"

"She's worth every penny," he said when I repeated this to him. "Please keep going."

I held that recipe to my heart. *Beautiful, funny, stuff.* I liked the order of it, the breadth of it. I was in a country of fertile hills carpeted in Indian paintbrush and pine forests, a place of nooks for dozing, making love, and the odd ruby unearthed in the fields. A country he'd invented, and we inhabited alone.

Ireland, I decided. And then forgot all about my game of nationalities.

First love at forty-four years of age. Sweet with words and jokes and cuddling. Complicated by histories of broken lives, starting over, difficult jobs, distance, his son's yawning depression, my yawning curiosity about myself, him, the us of us.

Such honey.

Such rue.

And then it was over. His work turned brutal, his son absorbed what was left of him, and I tried to get as small and unimposing as possible. His calls grew more infrequent, with stories I didn't understand about work, something involving Internet access. We discussed whether it was fair to me, the months he knew this project would gobble up. Neither of us wanted to break up but neither did he, quite, want to be together. I left the question of us to the bruised silence of deep space.

In the occasional moments of cold lucidity, I added another requirement in a boyfriend:

- Even if it's rhetorical and insincere, when a man calls he must say, "How are you?"

In the occasional moments of worldly humor about the non-situation, I formulated the Fourth Law. Men can't multitask. Every day I heard my colleague, Anna, through our office wall, dealing with her parents' doctors' appointments, her niece's genius, her sister's pregnancy, her wedding plans, her fiancé's family calendar. Anna did her job like clockwork. Women can multitask an infinite variety of necessities and scheduling, along with a career and remembering the dry cleaning. Men are good for two or maybe three items at a time. The Boy in Connecticut had work and trying to both love and curb his son who was well on his way to becoming a complete Dudley Dursley. A third item, like a girlfriend ninety minutes away, and he wasn't *There* anymore.

"I would add one thing," Dr. Miller said to this. "Sometimes there's no there, 'there.' " And this was the Fifth Law.

The winter droned on. A Sunday of low gray skies came, Valentine's Day approaching. I knew my boyfriend could care less but my parents did. I went into the neighborhood emporium of clever and tender artifacts. Eartha Kitt was singing and I smiled. It was a rare good moment. Witty cards and witty music, a good deed for my parents as I ran errands as though my heart was not cracking my rib cage, cozy in my very own neighborhood where I knew the clerks and had rapports that were fond and familiar.

Ugly struck as Barbara Cook began singing "This Nearly Was Mine." My hand hovered over a heart-studded card. The only time I ever saw my father cry was when Rossano Brazzi sang this song into an island night. It would arrest me anytime. That day it was the sweetest and sharpest possible slug on the jaw. I was buying a Valentine's Day card for my elderly parents when I wanted only to see the man I loved. I will never see him again, I mouthed silently to myself in the unwinding of the song. I was alone with the haunt of him. This was going to hurt wicked-bad.

In the Bat Cave, on the street, in the office, among the Stepfords, in but not of the general flow of humanity, I was 158 pounds of pain. I'd cracked 160 at last but I had nothing except a badly chapped nose to show for it. My immigration application, not to a member country of the United Nations, but to the magical places I'd once used food to take me—Narnia or the Secret Garden or Galleons Lap—hadn't been refused. It had been lost in bureaucratic shuffle.

14

GIRL

OVERBOARD

I *love you, Frances Kuffel,* he'd said the last night we spent together. I repeated it to myself with a twist that ran from my esophagus to my heart. *You're beautiful, you're funny, I like your stuff.*

And I'm smart and thin and I'll wait in silence forever if you ask, I argued and promised back to the silence of him. *How can you just stop?*

Grief was a form of bulimia. I took to listening to the music of high school, long years of crushes on boys who thought I was fun, maybe, in German class or a play rehearsal, but who went out with girls, thin and pink, on the weekends. "Wild World," "Car on a Hill," "So Far Away." Anything could unglue me. I broke down over spilled coffee beans, I got on trains that took me to Williamsburg instead of Midtown, I was almost unbeatable at my favorite computer game, and I slept, a little, with the help of six Sominex at a time.

Anna, my office colleague twenty years my junior and twenty years smarter in affairs of the heart, shook her head. "He's your first boyfriend, Frances. This is completely normal. Trust me. We've all been through it."

"Yeah, when you were sixteen. It's no wonder you're supposed to do this when you're sixteen. What else do you have to do when you're sixteen besides lie on the floor and cry? I'm forty-five, I can't afford this. I'll get my pants dirty. They're cashmere."

"He's a mess, Fran," Dr. Miller said. "The next time he emails, don't read it."

Yeah. Right.

Alix shut her office door and sat down to wait as I struggled to breathe. "Stay close to your pain," she said. "It's a sign of how hard you worked."

As if I had a choice.

"It's the addict's brain, going over the same thing again and again," Bridget said. "We get stuck in a loop. You remind me of how obsessive I used to be."

Glad I could help.

"Six to eight months," Jennifer speculated. "It took me a year to get over that bastard but I was out of control with food, with sugar. Although antidepressants helped."

Six months. That meant July. I felt like an infantile, half-dead nitwit of an alien as I asked questions like "How long does it take to get over a breakup?"

.   .   .

It was the Sunday phone call to my parents, each week the same conversation. How's the office, how's the diet, how's the weight, how's the boyfriend? Lately, I gnashed my teeth at it. I had depended on these calls over the years as the one source of understanding and succor I could count on. I wished, that week, that I had the kind of problems Mother and Daddy could fix, with 7-Up and antibiotics, a cool hand on my forehead. As February soldiered into March, it got harder to talk, to them or anyone else. The savor had gone out of my days. I missed him like salt. Nothing I did differentiated itself from anything else, so there was no answer to "How's the office?" "How are you?" prompted the taste of ashes on my tongue.

"What's new?" my father asked when he took the phone from Mom. The sound of his voice was the sound of imminent practicality, in which logical progressions could always be found, whether it's making French bread or getting over a breakup.

"Nothing," I said dully. "What's new with you?" Mom had already filled me in on the complacent week they'd spent, his reading and boxing matches, her quilting, their bridge group. But there was the chance he'd have a piece of politics he wanted to tell me about, or a new dinosaur theory. Anything to fill up our voids: his growing blindness, my lack of interest in anything at all.

"The usual," he said. "Are you dating?"

"I suppose."

"What does that mean?"

I sniffed loudly. "I don't know. I've talked to a few men. One took me to dinner at a nice Mexican restaurant this week."

"Really?" A window flew open in his voice. Daddy always wants to hear about New York restaurants. "Whadja have?"

"I don't remember." I scrunched my nose trying to recall the meal, the man's face. My bifocals pushed up and the room went as blurry as that evening. "Mole sauce, I think. I remember corn. Chicken?"

That I couldn't repeat the composition of a meal was a bad sign indeed. On the other hand, I had come to remember occasions less for what I ate than what I wore. That night was Harris tweed and a brick-red Michael Kors sweater.

"Are you going to see him again? He took you someplace nice. You should see him again."

"He didn't make me laugh. None of them make me laugh, Daddy." A wail was building along my rib cage, coiling up like the roller coaster at Coney Island before it whooshes its screaming cargo down.

He waited to get my attention for what he had to say in reply. "Has it occurred to you that there are more important things in a relationship besides laughing?"

It was my turn to pause, unsure of what to think. My sense of humor, irreverent and raunchy, is my father's legacy to me. For him to remove laughter from the recipe of love was a betrayal.

"We had other stuff," I said defensively of my Boy in Connecticut. "We . . ." I paused again. "We both like salad. We like to read." It was a paltry list. I couldn't tell my father what it was like when the Boy smiled at me as we made love, how his eyes had sunbursts at the corners because he smiled so intently, really looking at me, really *seeing* me, and how he'd stop a moment just to look and whisper, "You're beautiful, Frances Kuffel." It was like full dawn after a week of rain. I had been left to remember this stuff for both of us, double-duty mourning. "We have things in common," I finished lamely.

"Except he's gone."

You want sympathy, look for it between shit and syphilis in the dictionary.

"Yes."

"You better get busy, kid."

"I'm trying." The sob hit my throat. "I missed forty years," my voice cracked. "Everyone I went to school with is married or published or has tenure." I slid from my chair to the floor as I toiled to new peaks of martyrdom. "I'm so lonely, Daddy."

"I know, honey," he relented. "I want more than anything to see you with someone before—"

He stopped, cleared his throat. I cleared mine as well. We let it hang.

I wished I watched golf on television or had a new custard recipe to tell him about. I was tired of being Johnny-One-Note. "I feel like such a fake. My body is a wreck from being fat. I feel ashamed talking to men when I know what I really look like. What can I give them? I couldn't have children even if . . ."

It was a conversation of incomplete sentences.

If I found someone who could love me.

"You're depressed, kid. It's time for Prozac."

I resisted a moment. Hadn't I lost weight so I'd never need Prozac again? Thirty seconds later I was comforted. Jennifer had talked about antidepressants when she broke up with her last boyfriend. There was alleviation out there. I'd taken Prozac before; I knew that it offered a fresh start every morning, the remains of yesterday left in yesterday. I called my doctor the next morning.

The Prozac, at the lowest dose on a one-month prescription from my internist, let me notice the world beyond my bed and the Bat Cave a little. There came a brief Friday email about how much he hated his job and his son's noble attempt not to be disappointed because Dad had to miss a weeknight Scout meeting again. I replied that he was a good man and a good father. *If that's the last thing I ever say to him, I wished him luck,* I thought. *It's good karma to go out on. I could end it here.*

The Sixth Law About Men is that single men with children aren't single.

I went home to listen to David Gray sing "Say Hello Wave Goodbye" and then on to the jeering horns in Bartók's Concerto for Orchestra for good measure, deleted his emails, and substituted a friend's phone number on automatic dial. What few things—razor, toothbrush—he'd left in the Bat Cave I put in a shoebox, such a meager showing that I added others. The partner of a ruby earring I lost the first night we were together. The photos of us that my sister-in-law had hung copies of in her kitchen. No one recognized me in them, she had written. No one had ever seen me that happy. They hadn't recognized me after losing 170 pounds, either. The sum of his effect on me was a physical change as dramatic as 170 pounds. I sat down a moment to take it in, then tossed the last Kleenex I intended to cry into over him into the box.

I'd been disappointed in love when I was fat, but it was the grief of miscarriage, a deformed possibility of mostly unadmitted love that couldn't survive gestation. This was a funeral for an infant. It had a name and a personality and a future. And it was dead.

I found the book he'd given me for my birthday and added it to the box. The box had some heft now. I wanted my apartment to have no evidence left.

I'd fought too hard to be right where I was, fought too hard not to appreciate the irony. Heartbreak as an achievement—go figure! I'd never expected that "thin" would equal "happy." I just didn't count on being inhuman with pain as part of becoming a girl. That night, as I considered how to dispose of this coffin that held the best I'd ever been, I weighed 155 pounds, less in every way I could think of than he'd ever seen me.

I had no plot of land to bury us in, no fireplace to burn us, no pond to pitch us into. If I put us in the trash downstairs, we'd hang around until Monday, directly beneath my bed, a thing I couldn't risk. I decided to take the shoebox to the Promenade, the long park that faces downtown Manhattan. It was full of gawkers who'd come to look at the light beams where the World Trade Center towers had been six months ago. I got a couple of odd looks when I placed the box in the trash; they must have thought I was dumping the corpse of my beloved Chihuahua.

It was over. The pear trees along Montague Street were in ghastly blossom. Holy Week was approaching.

I had deleted his email address, rewritten the Filofax page, and substituted another phone number on speed dial. Communication would now have to be an effort. I wouldn't bump into him in my home anymore. I was clearly—*cleanly*—alone.

I did not feel clean. I was angry at the betrayal of my thinitude. I was lonely and made lonelier by the humorless Matchdot dates I endured. It was appropriate that we were heading into the solemnities of Good Friday.

"Boy, do I have a whole new appreciation for the gospels," I told my brother.

"Oh?" Caution fought curiosity in his response. Jim was fervently fundamentalist, and he knew from experience that in questions of religion I was liable to say anything. "How so, Sis?"

"I've always found Jesus to be kind of a dope. I'm not interested in the afterlife and I resent the liturgy for saying we pray for things *through* Jesus. He's more of a secretary than a divinity." There was a pained silence. Jim was probably bracing himself for a riff on Christ's homosexual harem. "But I've been walking around in a state of 'my God, my God, why hast thou forsaken me?' "

"Matthew 42:46," he said as automatically as "gesündheit."

"Whatever. God is gone."

"You know, Francie, when Christ accused God of abandoning Him, God really had. As hard as it was to turn His back on His son, He had to. Christ had to die alone, without His father and without turning away from His father."

Not bad, I thought, *for a man whose minister fixes small appliances during the week.* Then the enormity of what he'd said hit with a *whomp.* "I'm scared, Jimmie. I'm alone and I'm scared."

"Go find God, Sis. *Go out.* Look for him. *Find* Him."

I sighed. God knows I'd done yeoman's work at talking to God that winter. I'd obeyed Bridget's rule of gratitude, getting down on my knees morning and night to thank Him for the material and intellectual gifts at my disposal. I'd tried pleading with Him. I'd tried praying for the Boy, saying, "I don't care what you do to me, but please let him be safe and loved." I'd tried shaking my fist at the pewter winter skies with demands: "Make him call, make him *remember.*" I gave eighty dollars to the diocesan fund-raising drive because the bishop promised to pray for our intentions. "Bless Dudley Dursley," I wrote on the form. I knew what I was asking. Dudley was a food addict as surely as I was, filling up the unfillable with anything he could put in his mouth when Dad and the few other people in his life inevitably could not give enough love to sate him. Dudley would either molder in his addiction or he would have to learn to find love wherever he could, like radio telescopes sweeping the heavens for errant alien broadcasts. I had done both. I'd curled into the food until I disappeared, and I'd learned, sometimes, to seek out the blessings of being alive and human. From the Stepfords, from the lucky sighting of a man feeding his parrot an ice cream cone on Montague Street, from the horrible opportunities thin had thrown at me.

"Help Dudley find his way to happiness."

Silence, from Connecticut and from heaven. Both of my

gods' answering machines had filled up and I was talking to dial tones.

It was time to try a different kind of talking.

On Palm Sunday the church bulletin announced parish penance. There would be a service of prayer and reflection, and confession.

I cast back to my last confession, before confirmation when I was fourteen. Twenty-nine years. How many times had I taken the Lord's name in vain since then, for Christ's sake? I was guilty of the seven deadly sins on a daily basis. And I hated God.

I had a lot to confess.

Assumption is a good church to make penance in. The only dogmas the Roman Catholic Church has ever settled on are the unbreachable truths of the virgin birth and the bodily assumption of the Virgin Mary into heaven. The interior, reflecting the name and the theme of the Assumption, is delicate and feminine. The altar is dominated with the Virgin in serene prayer for us sinners, bookended on each side with statues of the Holy Family and St. Theresa of the Little Flowers. You have to look around for the suffering of Christ. It felt safe.

Assumption's two confessionals filled quickly. I found myself in the sacristy, face-to-face with a jolly priest I'd never, thankfully, met.

"Do I do the 'Bless me, Father, for I have sinned' thing? I don't think I remember it anymore." We laughed. "It's been twenty-nine years since my last confession," I added, the next words in the docket of admissions. Next to follow would be "and these are my sins," venial on to mortal. And I thought I couldn't remember?

"Look, Father, I've committed every sin in the book except for some of the really big ones. No murder, no grand larceny, no adultery. But everything else, lots and lots."

"Why don't we talk about what's weighing on you, then?"

"I hate God."

"Ah."

"He let me be born and He didn't . . . My birth mother got pregnant in 1956 and would have or should have had an abortion but she didn't or couldn't. I was born by mistake and God let it happen but He hasn't taken any responsibility for it. He let me slip through the cracks but that's it, that's as far as His gig goes. As soon as I do or get something good, it falls apart. I got good parents, but I got fat. I got thin, and I'm more miserable than ever. I'm on my own. And I hate God."

The priest sat back in his chair and chuckled. Actually, I think priests must hear versions of this frequently. All anyone really wants to know is that one is loved, unconditionally. Priests are the masters of ceremonies of that love. There at baptism, there for extreme unction, sanctifying puberty and marriage and penitence in between. He'd probably heard this a hundred times.

"Have you read Jeremiah?"

"Not recently."

"Ah. Well, you're not alone. Jeremiah calls God a rapist. The Bible is full of rage against God. God is there to be raged against."

"Aren't I supposed to love Him, even when He's a son of a bitch?" My head dropped in weariness. "I'm tired, Father. I'm so tired."

"Of what?"

"Fighting. Fighting myself. Fighting Him. Fighting to love Him. Fighting when He's gonna win anyway. The Our Father and that bunk about 'thy will be done'? As if I have a choice. He's God, right? He's pretty much going to do whatever He wants, whether I pray or not. He's always gonna win. So here I am and I pretty much hate myself. Is that His will? Is that what He's going to win, the day I finally give in to hating myself once and for all?"

"Think a little more about the Lord's Prayer. Think about the golden rule. 'Love thy neighbor as thyself.' Jesus didn't demand that we love God; He told us to ask for help and to love each other—and *ourselves*. Think about that. Hating yourself violates the golden rule as much as hurting your next-door neighbor."

We talked for an hour. He told me to say three Our Fathers and suggested I might want to make another confession before twenty-nine years slipped by again.

The crocuses danced their purple and saffron braggadocio, freesia and dogwood were in soft-focus bloom as I walked home. I'd gotten out and squared something. Maybe not with God—did I really even believe in all that?—but with the past that the rite and the Church and prayers represented that evening. I had talked about the queered bargains I'd struck with God, or with myself if there was no God. I felt a little bouncier. I'd met with sympathy when I said some outrageous things— things, I grinned, I could have been burned at the stake for saying six hundred years ago. Glory be, I had the distinct impression that God's master of ceremonies had felt the same outrage himself. Odd that Jim, the brother I had habitually ignored, had a part in getting me there. Odd, really, wasn't it, that I kept finding help, kept finding *friends*, when I announced my need of it?

I called Jennifer the next day. I needed Stepfords who had fallen in love and been crushed by it, who had survived long enough to make raucous fun of it and who would tell me what to do next. She invited me to dinner with Christy. They were professional daters. I knew they'd know the deal.

. . .

"It's good, Frances," Jennifer said. "You're feeling your feelings."

God, it was hackneyed, this twelve stepese, the pidgin English between the language of the Planet of Fat, where feelings
are solvable in a fast two thousand calories, and Earth English,
in which humans are accustomed to feelings because they've
been having them all along, on schedule. I was equally sick of
twelve stepese being right.

"That's all I've been doing," I answered bitterly.

"No, it's not," Christy objected. She was Jennifer's best
friend among the Stepfords, with twenty years' experience of
not having six sizes of clothes in her closet. "You haven't eaten
over it."

"You don't cry through meetings anymore, either," Jennifer
added. "Remember last month? You were a wreck. Now you
can talk about it without falling apart. That's called progress,
Miss Thing. It's time to enjoy yourself again. See your friends,
go to the movies. Get laid. You look mah-vell-ous. I wish I was
as thin as you."

I pushed the carcass of my chicken away and sat back to
study them. Christy and Jennifer knew exactly what they were
doing with men. Christy was engaged to a snowy-haired blue-
suede-shoes Elvis, with no intention of marrying him until he
got his shit together, and with no intention of letting anyone but
herself decide when his shit was gathered. In her mid-fifties, she
was blond, elfin, and had the energy of a woman who has not
settled for second best. I admired her ability to live with a thesis. And there was Jen, younger than I by thirteen years, small
as a mobile rocket and twice as lethal. Construction workers

followed her and it was no wonder, with her low-slung, hippy walk, showing skin at every possible gap in her clothing. I admired her nakedness. By contrast, I looked like an extra in *The Prime of Miss Jean Brodie*.

She gazed back at me. There was admiration in her look as well. "Got it, darling? You've just passed the initiation test for the Brooklyn Sluts and Supper Club. You got dumped. You're horny and you think your life is pointless without a man, no matter how important you tell yourself your work is. It's OK. We've all been there. We get used to being pointless and go about our business again."

So it's a sixteen-year-old's heartbreak, I thought as I looked at her hard, smiling, obsidian eyes, at Christy's elfish grin. That didn't mean they didn't respect it as genuine. I had one more thing in common with girls. I'd live through it. I had known all along I would but oh, God, when would I be passing for alive again, let alone human and girly?

"It's essential to finish losing the weight," Bridget said the morning I reported my weight. One hundred and forty-six pounds. "Now you have to begin living life on life's terms." What did she think I'd been doing?

Once again I had to take stock of this body. It had shivered and grieved itself beyond my expectations of thinitude. It was alive, this body, even if my heart was still so sore it could make me blink in surprise at a lurch of uninvited memory. I could let it dictate life's terms for a while.

The discomfort I'd gone through when I got down to about 220 pounds returned. My tailbone was sore from sitting, the insides of my knees ached when I slept on my side. I could see the ribs in my upper chest. I could pull up a thick sheet of skin off my stomach when I was lying down. It was equal parts repelling and fascinating, this latest science experiment with my body.

Go out. My brother's words mingled with Bridget's. *Live life on life's terms.*

I went to the gym and discovered this body had the energy of hibernation, the insistence of betrayal, the restlessness of waiting for spring. It was good to feel my body again—the sweat and cold dry throat, the muscles warming in my legs, the floating peace when I left. Like the simplicity of my food plan that had dropped the last ten pounds without my noticing, I could *do* this. I could walk out my front door and go to the gym.

I was homesick. Six weeks earlier I felt hollow from the missing of him; now it was the calm of Flathead and the Rockies that I missed. I wanted egress into my mountains. I pushed the treadmill's incline up to seven and thought about the mountains. I wanted to be ready to try whatever I wanted to try.

I wanted to be a different Frances than the girl who'd headed to Metro-North every weekend. I wanted to be unrecognizable to him, flinty and unhurtable.

"I want to stop traffic," I told my friend, Shirley Qian, as we sorted through racks of clothes in her shop. She smiled slyly and reached for a pile of slinky sweaters. "No, no," I hastened. "I don't want to stop traffic because I'm hot-looking. I want to stop it because the traffic is afraid *not* to stop." Her smile changed to conniving as she pulled a mean little pinstripe off the rack. I wanted to be elegant, unassailable, stern.

I left wearing one of Shirley's short skirts and my leather jacket. I walked across a Saturday-thronged SoHo, feeling strong and rangy. All in black I was, unforgiving Doc Martens and a heavy ribbed cotton turtleneck, taking no prisoners as I strode along, crossing against lights and glaring at drivers. Women were looking, noticing; I noticed their notice. Their assessment was an itemized list. My black clothes, my face; then my legs, earrings, the shopping bag.

Wasn't this what and who I had wanted to be, two and a half years ago when I arrived on Earth and began measuring myself against neighborhoods? To pass as a native. Men were looking with reserved admiration. I was pretty, but I was also Teflon-safe in my black defined clothes. I looked like a woman loping off to the West Side subway with big things on her mind.

If only, I thought, *I was.*

I'm one of the lucky ones in the voyage to the Planet of Girls. I had a destination; I knew what I was setting out to accomplish once I arrived. I wasn't naïve enough to think it would be an easy stroll across the universe, but I had a direction nonetheless. I forgot to ask about the aftermath of success: *then what?*

"First you got the body you always wanted," the Good Doctor Miller explicated, thinking it out as she said it. "And then you got the body you didn't know you wanted." No one else seemed to want my body, either.

But she was right. I hadn't planned for this body. My categories were as fucked up as they'd been that day Tethys droned on about her party in the Hamptons and I'd looked around to see I'd been dropped from my tribe of fat people. I'd set my rocket ship's course for thin-as-in-normal and landed on a drifting continent.

Finishing is not success.

Can you finish a body? What's the point? It wasn't like I wanted to enter a bodybuilding competition; I wasn't going snowboarding anytime soon. I'd run out of money for shopping.

I hadn't thought what it would be like to be thinner than I'd been for three years, but it had always been there, a possibility, touched when I'd been on IVs. Once upon a time, I'd bottomed

out on food and the limitations of obesity. Now I'd bottomed
out on dieting and the appalling infinities that being thin offered.
It had the flat thud of taking one more step on a staircase that's
already ended. I was safely on my feet, nothing was overtly
wrong, I had only to keep walking. But some tiny fiber in my inner ear was shivering and I quaked as I took up my pace again,
my balance off.

I wanted something, I didn't know what, didn't know where
I could find it. My mountains were three thousand miles away.
I was a castaway.

From grief to relieved mania to empty.

It had been a tiring week of meetings and lunches with foreign agents and publishers, capped by a party for literary agents
on Friday evening. I knew what was coming—Alix had yet to
remain sober in a setting with an open wine bottle—but I could
not know that my past was about to catch up with me.

Already tipsy, Alix assaulted my old boss, Barbara, with a
hearty greeting, then returned with another glass of wine for instant replays. "I just stuck my hand out and said, 'How *are* you,
Barbara? You must be having a good book fair with number
one on the best-seller list!' She was in shock—heh-heh-heh." I
laughed feebly along with her. "I *stuck* my hand out!" Alix
started in again.

You can always tell a publishing party by the mountain of
book bags at the coat rack. I wanted to climb into that pile. I
stayed in the corner of the loft room, near the crudités, avoid-
ing Barbara and her daughter as I always did at functions. I did
not like making pleasantries with my past.

"Now," Alix announced, "go mingle!"

Back to the crudités trays where I snarfed raw cauliflower

and carrots and exchanged no-talk about the hors d'oeuvres, hoping it looked like mingling. Later, trying to divorce myself from the food, I went out to the terrace and let the wind off the Hudson smoke my cigarette. The party was winding down. Alix and I were among the last to gather up our bags, but not until she tried to get me to jitterbug to the Glenn Miller, loud in the nearly empty room, on the CD player. Lucky for me, I didn't know how to jitterbug. Unlucky for the security guard because she forced him into a turn or two.

I was limping in my mules by the time we got to the street. The bright May evening swam around me like the first warning of a flu bug as Alix went through the catalogue of people she'd talked to, what she'd said or teased them about. I winced, from my shoes and from her stories. Alix got giggly with wine, weirdly flirtatious with a combative, dictatorial edge to it. Tipsy and flighty as she was, I was afraid she'd fly off in a gust of wind if I didn't find her a taxi, and Eleventh Avenue was bumper-to-bumper as I laughed and prayed for a cab. Success came two long blocks east. We kissed goodbye, wished each other a good weekend; I hailed my own cab and gave directions to the Heights, easing back to wriggle my toes at last.

The sunset-gilded streets flashed by as an isn't-this-what-I-always-imagined moment washed over me. Wasn't the week of lunches and the party the Marlo Thomas/Mary Tyler Moore fantasy I'd come to New York for?

We zipped from Eleventh Avenue through Washington Square, down Broadway and the City Hall buildings, a fast review of the sixteen years I'd been one body, fat or thin, among zillions of others, anonymous, pushing against loneliness. The Javits Center would always remind me of Barbara—*you big baby!*—and of Dennis, who lived on Thirty-fourth Street. I hadn't seen him for months and I missed him. Chelsea, great restaurants and shoe stores, Henry Holt country, and the compromise destination for Penguin lunches. I'd taught four nights a week for ten years in Chelsea, trying to hammer the difference between "its" and "it's" into minds occupied with hockey and getting laid. NYU—*you flunked out, didn't you,* I sneered at myself. *Didn't notice the calendar and presto! you had a Middle English final you hadn't studied for.* Lower Broadway, Little Italy, Chinatown—afternoons and evenings of walking-and-talking with friends long gone. City Hall. The fountain where the Boy from Connecticut and I had kissed such a long kiss that I could probably find our shadows seared into the concrete like the immolated citizens of Hiroshima.

Years of Entenmann's, pushing—the wrong way, but pushing—to get right here, my crowning achievement in being able to buy and wear Dolce & Gabbana, go home to the Bat Cave which was waiting silently in perpetual dark. *Congratulations, Frances. You're a real New Yorker at last.* The season finale of *Sex and the City,* a Gershwin song, a Wasserstein plot.

The weekend stretched and grumbled like a grizzly bear waking up in spring, slow but hungry, ready to take me down. It was Friday. In ten minutes I would be able to kick off my pinching shoes, put on shorts, and—what?

Maybe I'd run out and get a hobby, or maybe they delivered? Maybe tonight I should write my masterpiece, or vacuum behind the bookcases, or take a walk on my crenulated feet to the piers or Carroll Gardens, or finally watch *Berlin Alexanderplatz?*

I was too weary to be useful or even to amuse myself.

How had I done it all those years?

I'd given everything away. My brain, my heart, my body. I was down to my soul, a pathetic flaccid balloon of no color, left in a corner years after the party had ended.

Thud.

The staircase had already given out.

That evening the best I could do was to love an insane man who once loved me back. I found his office website in Connecticut and I emailed him. He'd written a month earlier, saying he missed talking to me. Talking: a good thing. It was not my body he missed but our way of conversation, the play of minds. It was safe, two minds with lots of words. The flare of triumph I'd had when he'd written in April turned to hope that better than nothing actually was better than nothing. I was finished. I wanted to go home.

Once upon a time I had commented that he and I were better together than we were apart, that we challenged each other to be better.

I wanted to be better.

Once upon a time he noted how perfectly we puzzled together in sleep.

I wanted to sleep.

Once upon a time he stood in Grand Central Station telling me a story of the tiny snowmen we would build on his porch railing.

I wanted a new story.

Maybe, I wrote, we could see if we could try again.

And then I began to eat.

15

AN ALIEN VISITOR
TO THE PLANET OF WOMEN

I was eating. Oatmeal, my fallback food, sweet and mouth-filling. Deli chicken with its rich skin and dripping fat. Brown rice with salsa and black olives. "Abstinent" food, but I was sick from it and gaining weight. It turned off the goblins in my head for the duration of the eating and the duration of the stomachache.

"Are you purging?" my psychiatrist, Dr. Rosenblatt, asked.

"I wish."

Doctors and shrinks take eating disorders seriously when toilets are involved. Bingeing and living with the consequences—the spiking body temperature, stomach so full that my surgical scars stung and wept, the aches deep in my flesh, the twenty-pound weight gain in a week—didn't rate highly in the psychiatric community. I invoked losses, going for the 188-pound version, winning my point. There was an impressive silence.

"You lost a part of your self."

It was my turn to pause. What had Fredi said when she saw me a couple of years ago? *Frances, you're half your size. You lost half of yourself.* I'd heard it a lot, always with the word "size." Dr. Rosenblatt came down hard on "self."

"Maybe. It was my evil Siamese twin but we were used to each other. At least I was never alone."

Unlike the Good Doctor Miller, my psychiatrist was very thin. She wanted to explore what this notion of the loss of self involved, yet another undiscovered country. I was less inclined toward indulgence. Maybe I used depression to re-create the Planet of Fat. It accomplished the same thing. I was small in depression, I was all-important in it. I was the star of my own show.

She wrote a prescription for Zoloft and I wrote her a hefty check. We agreed to do it again in a month.

The emails between the Boy from Connecticut and me trickled out. On the Fourth of July I found myself tirelessly pushing leg weights at the gym. Ninety pounds for fifty reps, then a hundred and ten pounds. Seesaw, seesaw, breathe in, breathe out. My mind lifted out of my brainpan to a white place, thirty thousand feet in clouds, tranquil, mesmerizing. I was taken aback to feel tears rolling down my cheeks. I'd let myself get simple and the last wad of sorrow and self-blame had crested. Maybe I wasn't worth it to him, or maybe he couldn't have moved his son and his attachment to solitude and panic aside for any woman. It didn't matter. I stopped and rested my forehead against my knees as I cried out the last of it.

Number Seven in the Laws About Men: never try to get back together with someone who's already broken your heart. He knows exactly how to break it again.

With silence, with not showing up, with excuses.

A few weeks later, as the Zoloft began to lift my cocktail hour existential crisis, a man from the dating service the Good Doctor Miller told me to join called. He took me to lunch at a midtown restaurant where he'd made reservations. He'd been struck by the way I answered the service's questionnaire, "Is it important that your companion share your religion?" "No," I wrote, "but it would be nice if he got the jokes." He did.

On our third or fourth date, I kissed *him* goodbye. Chastely. As I would a friend. But it was a kiss, and I did it.

Apologetically, the Catholic Boy explained the Eighth Law About Men. Men are attracted to a face and a body first. "It doesn't mean anything," he said as we walked along Second Avenue. I was enjoying the warm night. He, apparently, was enjoying the bare-legged women enjoying the warm night. "We're men. We *look*. It doesn't mean we want, but we *look*." I took satisfaction in the Eighth Law. The Catholic Boy had looked at me and he wanted to see me again.

He also confirmed a thing I had long suspected was true, the

Ninth Law: men learn quickly (give credit where credit is due—in an afternoon or in the course of a half dozen evenings) to like what they find beautiful. "I didn't think I was girlfriend material," I explained of my sparse romantic history.

He laughed, a rare, creaky laugh I liked more and more. "Why wouldn't you be? You're pretty, you're smart, you're nice."

The Catholic Boy asked me out the second time because I was pretty, but he asked me out on the seventh or eighth date because of the other adjectives. Adjectives I earned in obesity.

I was beginning to understand the old saying that women find increasing beauty in the man they've already come to like.

It had been two years since I'd seen the mountains and my extended family. My homesickness was growing, and my parents, Lisa, and my brother reported plaintively that they were homesick for me. After a battle with Alix to take a long weekend, I booked a flight to Kalispell, bought a couple bags of sugar-free almond bark and peanut butter cups, and skied off to confront my parents' increasing decrepitude and the test of what I had achieved on the treadmill.

I woke to rain my first day at Flathead, but the sky cleared by midmorning. It was a shock after the grayed sepia of New York in a heat wave. I moved gingerly from my parents' dining room to the deck overlooking the garnet lake, sick from eating all the so-called sugarless chocolates the day before. I shook out a cigarette and promised myself I would leave the remaining turtles and peanut butter cups for the family. *Start over today,* I thought as I watched whitecaps riffing the water. *You'll have a normal breakfast and get on with it,* I lectured myself as I tied on my sneakers for the trip Lisa and I had planned for that morning.

But I knew exactly where the chocolates were.

Lisa brought her usual charge of energy with her, debating, as she bomped in, whether we should hike the Garden Wall at Logan Pass or a pretty trail through cedars. "Do you want views or easy walking, Francie?" she was plotting before she reached the kitchen. I was unwrapping Stilton and brie to add to the platter of pepperoni and smoked turkey. We'd wanted a day in Glacier Park through the years of my thinitude, but it never happened. As it was, this was stealing a day from my parents. I opened a bag of rosemary potato chips and helped myself before offering it to her. Lisa looked at me, saw my mouth set in the determination to eat, and took a handful, turning to double-check that my parents would watch Sophie while we went for our hike.

They were good sports about our plans to leave at seven the next morning. They'd always been supremely generous, with their home and their money, with their faith in me. Eating taffy, I leaned over my father's chair. He sat in the full sun of the picture window with an enormous magnifying glass and two strong Ott lights, poring over a photograph of my office staff as I screamed the names of faces he eked out one at a time.

He looked up at me and smiled. "I couldn't remember if you came out for Christmas. I knew you must have because of the clock you gave me."

Having taught us where to find sympathy, my father wasn't looking for it from me. He knew his body was winding down, an organ at a time: his heart, his eyes, his hearing, his prostate, the part of his brain that housed Christmas and names. There was no regret in his voice about biology but there was a deep hole where he couldn't remember *me*. I knew it because he was talking about it. He didn't say much about the disappointments of losing his body—it was age, he understood that. At eighty-five, he figured he'd had a good run of it.

We were closer in biology at that moment than he knew. I

was losing my body as he talked about the things he found hard to remember, diverting my fears of his and Mother's accumulating losses with thoughts of ice cream and cinnamon toast. Anything not to think about what might come next for them. I wanted to run like a yellow-bellied coward back to Brooklyn. At the same time I wondered if I should move into the guesthouse to care for them.

He talked about his interests, soldiering on as he continued to do as many of the things he used to as possible. So what if the petunias were planted a little oddly, he joked at my mother's sighing over the front garden her arthritis kept her out of. He'd even painted the deck of the guesthouse. When more finesse was called for, there was family to help. Lisa came out once a week from Kalispell to mow the lawn, and Jim came up from Missoula to help with repairs. I was wanted but not needed here, or needed for something I didn't have it in me to give. Unless I ate, unless I got so fat again that this would be the only place that would gather me in its arms.

Mom and Dad had always looked past my anger for the need and sad talents lurking under the fat. Sometimes, like the lake, they could swallow me whole. Or did I swallow them, along with every molecule of food I could wedge into myself, so that we were one and the same? Was I their portrait of Dorian Gray? It was the burden of doubt I carried, that I would swallow or smother those I loved most. Their recourse would be to go away from me. Had I done that to the Boy in Connecticut?

I had wanted to bring a boyfriend home to meet my parents. I wanted them to know that I would not be alone when they die. I had planned great adventures for my thin body: ballet class, fencing lessons, riding the Cyclone at Coney Island, wearing an evening gown for some well-lit occasion in lieu of the proms I didn't go to. I had done none of these things. I could not reassure them that I had love and a fulfilling, bright professional future.

"When you were little and too excited by being at the lake to nap," he said, handing the photographs back to me, "we'd take you out in the boat. You remember *Blue Boy*? You'd be asleep by the time we got to the point. You loved the lake more than anything."

"We should go over to Indian Bay," I said. "Take a look-see at the old stomping grounds." We'd rented a cabin there for years, the kids sorted into packs according to age, the parents playing poker all night, our Lab, Sandy, fishing for minnows and taking on that Chesapeake retriever we swore had rabies. "We had an amazing childhood." I patted his cheek and pulled his cool earlobe, such a funny bit of flesh, such a funny thing to show him my love.

"You're not angry anymore? About, you know, the teasing and . . . the things you didn't get to do?"

"No," I lied, searching for a bigger true thing than regret. "How could I, with you for a daddy?"

My daddy. My daddy who was in the recovery room when I came around from my tonsillectomy when I was four years old, murmuring the safest words I have ever heard: "Wake up, Francie. That's right. Wake up, wake up. Everything's OK. Wake up." My daddy who knew the names of constellations and mountains he couldn't see any more, knew what mushrooms were edible, passed gas for seventy-two hours straight during the Battle of Pork Chop Hill, who built a sailboat and resoled my clown doll's feet and made enamel teapot earrings at my request.

He was tickled silly by my weight loss, but I had wanted him to know I wouldn't be alone.

And I couldn't.

So I ate.

It was a classic spiral, one I had managed not to do in my four years among the Stepfords. From the sex of cheese, sausage, cherries, "sugarless" candy, I boogied on to my mother's cherry

cobbler, and from there to the peanut butter cookies and snick-
erdoodles she made for the grandchildren. White flour—sugar—
yee-haw! I was sneaking at first, then eating apologetically, then
blatantly. "Well, if I'm gonna do it," I told Mom, "I might as
well get it out of my system." She agreed but she was worried,
too. Later I overheard my father asking what happened to the
box of chocolate marshmallow cookies.

"There were twelve. I had two."

"I had one," she said.

"Francie ate the other nine?"

It was that eight-year-old moment when my mother had to
intercede for me—apologize, lie, ignore, dare him to blow up at
the truth.

"I guess so."

Great, I thought. *You're not only eight years old, out of control, sick to your stomach, and gaining weight, but you've deprived an eighty-five-year-old deaf and blind man of one of his
few treats, Wal-Mart's pinwheel cookies.*

I should have picked up several packages. At $1.89, we
could've all been happy.

A day later, I was not exactly making Lisa happy. I stopped to
catch my breath on the boardwalk that leads from the visitors'
center to the foot of Mount Oberlin at Logan Pass. I was already tuckering out, breathing hard and doubting whether I'd
be able to do this hike. This was supposed to be the easy part,
with its graded walkways. We were being passed right and left
by fatties in fanny packs and "I ♥ Grizzly Bears" T-shirts. Lisa
looked worried as I called for another stop. How much failure
had she agreed to witness if I couldn't even keep up with these

selves I used to be? I summoned another breath and gasped, "OK, let's go on." She sighed in answer, the sigh of patience. Lisa was always patient with me.

What would happen when we left the boardwalk for an actual trail?

She led, of course. It was pretty, this path toward Mount Reynolds, which she thought would get us headed toward Heavy Runner, a mountain we chose, on my first real hike, for its name. We were at tree line. The lodge poles were dwarves, shaggy and deep green, and there were aprons of Indian paintbrush, buttercups, and grass-widows. The sky was robin's egg blue and cloudless, the whooshing wind the only sound. It made me think of *Heidi*.

Two weeks earlier Lisa let her trail runner pals lure her up Reynolds and she was so scared she sat down in the middle of the climb and cried. It was an evil anvil of a mountain, *Picnic at Hanging Rock*, Mount Doom. It was calling us. Somehow she couldn't find the fork where we should have turned north and east to Heavy Runner. We pressed on and every once in a while I asked to take a break. I was no longer out of breath, I just needed to get stupid for a minute or two after walking across shifting seas of bouldery rocks followed by morning-stiff fields of snow. We were watching our feet so carefully that if we hadn't stopped we would have missed the sliver of St. Mary's through the saddle of Reynolds and Heavy Runner. I didn't know St. Mary's could be seen from Logan, I told her.

"You're doing good, Francie," she reassured me. "When I said bring your gym shoes I thought they'd be trail sneakers like mine, not workout sneakers. But you're doing really good. It'll be worth it, trust me."

We started up a slope of sliding shale fragments and her reassurances built. "You won't believe what we're going to see. Are you sure you're OK?"

I wanted her to turn around and listen. She wouldn't have

heard anything but the wind. I was slower and more wary in my steps than she, but I wasn't panting. I wasn't even breathing hard.

"Yep," I said, picking my way out of the scree and onto a steep hillock of bigger but equally unstable rocks. "That was the bad part, this is fine."

We told each other this for four hours—*that* was awful, we've got the difficult walking licked now. It was a complete lie, especially coming down when we both knew what was coming next, but it felt good to say it.

I couldn't believe what I saw when we breached one last saddle. Hidden Lake maybe a thousand feet down a vertical drop to the southwest, Jackson Glacier smearing another precipice across the valley of snow we saw mountain goat tracks in. It was . . .

It was all I ever wanted.

"Can you believe I'm doing this?" I asked. "Can you believe I have the breath to ask if you believe I'm doing this?"

"This is *not* my Auntie Francie," she said. "I could believe I had anybody else up here with me except you." She frumped her face in the glare of the sun. "Maybe ten percent of the people who come to the park see Hidden Lake. One percent see Jackson." She shook her head. "And you *smoke. And* you've been here for one day and you're climbing at seven thousand feet. I can't believe we're doing this."

"I love this," I said. These were the mountains of my life, which I was standing *on,* for Christ's sake. I loved the paintbrush that had passed from red to a coral I'd never seen, and rarely saw this late in the season. I'd used up my film, not knowing there were better views to come, and I was disappointed that the day was too short to keep going, the trip too brief to do another hike.

All I ever wanted was to be able to go where my eyes led me. All I ever wanted was to know that if I had the time I could go on and on. All I ever wanted was to belong. That day my niece led me up and in, to views and horizons. I belonged to her and I belonged to the mountains I grew up in.

We didn't find what Lisa called the "mouth of the lion," the first chute she crawled when she topped Reynolds. Nor did we get to Heavy Runner. But coming back down a two-foot-wide patch of scree, with Reynolds shouldering us on one side and the thousand-foot-drop on the other, she stopped in alarm at the skitter of pebbles behind her. She turned to see me sliding down the loose rock, on the sides of my sneakers, leaning into the incline of the mountain.

"Where'd you learn to do that, Franny?" she asked suspiciously.

"What?"

"Ski on the sides of your feet?"

"I dunno. Nowhere?"

We looked out over acres of snow far below, pristine except for the crisscross of mountain goat tracks. I was wondering how we could, if we had time, zig and zag our way down there. Lisa was speculating similar adventures because she broke the hollow-winded quiet by saying, "You know, I always say you're the intellectual aunt, the one who makes me read and think. I *get* why you were out of breath on the boardwalk. You were bored. Up here you have to think. You're fine as long as it's a puzzle." She laughed her driest, evilest laugh, one of our shared secrets that says we have secrets. "You are in *sooo* much trouble. I've got you figured out; you have no excuses now. You can hike anything if you can do this. Next year we're going overnight into Waterton. You won't *believe* what you'll see there."

I was sublimely happy as I slipped-slid through this patch we were sure was the worst. All I ever wanted was to have no excuses.

I got back to Brooklyn just after midnight on Wednesday. I weighed 182 pounds. I had done damage to myself. Over the next week, I brought it down to 171. I went to meetings Thursday, Friday, and Saturday. My food was rigid. I hedged about having been a little "wild" with it while I was away. Only to Jennifer, whose abstinence was uneven, did I tell the truth. Bridget was out of town for two weeks; I had time to debate whether to confess or decide that the intervening run of abstinence made up for bread and butter, cobbler, ice cream, cookies—the whole *shandeh un a charpeh*. I was looking for something.

At a noon meeting, a fatty, smug in her chub and new abstinence from white flour, said, "God wants me to be right where I am now. In this body, in this moment."

Maybe that's what I am looking for, the moment or God. Did God want me to eat a box of Wheat Thins in bed? No. Yes. What I did know was that if there was a God, and if He was a loving God, He loved me as I chain-ate crackers against the turmoil of being home. If there wasn't a God, an equally real possibility, then the job of loving the person in bed with Nabisco fell to me.

At least I was home. Brooklyn Heights, the fitful habitability of the Bat Cave, Anna at the office, the Stepfords, Starbucks, the gym, the doctors Miller and Rosenblatt, my food scale, Church of the Assumption, my computer, the N/R train, Pam, and Jennifer. And the Catholic Boy.

Montana was my soul but New York was my brian. I knew I would always be torn—between the two literal states, the metaphorical alien and human, between food and abstinence. Surviving the breakup with the Boy from Connecticut reinforced what I knew very well in my obesity. Even when my heart is busted, my mind is a busy, horrible, beautiful place.

I had a chance here, in New York, to be invisible or to be whatever I wanted to be, no matter what size I rocked in at.

Or almost invisible.

The Catholic Boy was fascinated by the story of my weight loss. Did guys look at me now? This is the Tenth Law About Men: men want to know if other men look at their women.

Who knew? I wasn't proficient at telling the difference between friendliness and flirtation—hadn't he noticed? And I was so inured to appalled second glances that the whole business of being looked at ricocheted right off me.

I was glad to have a story to report to him at last.

I was walking to Fifth Avenue at noon. Outside the Peninsula Hotel, I noticed a handsome sort of man hurrying in the opposite direction. He noticed me at the same moment that I noticed him: a casual, almost practical glance except that we weren't on a collision course, we were only making sure we weren't on a collision course. I looked again—women indulge some of the Laws, too—at the same moment that *he* looked again. It was one second of mutual interest, of admiration. I was wearing sunglasses, so he wasn't responding to my first, practical look, and couldn't see my second look. But I caught his head turning, sharply, as we passed each other.

"Guess who it was?" I challenged the Catholic Boy, sitting back and putting my feet comfortably up on the trashcan beneath my desk. "Come on, guess."

He was at a loss, of course, but he was laughing with me; I

think he liked my enjoyment. I think he knew I had put my feet up and was offering myself, rich as apple pie, to his appetite.

"I don't know. Bill Clinton?"

"Eric Clapton," I informed him. "Eric fucking Clapton gave *me* a double take. You're definitely paying for dinner tonight."

Bridget was not indulgent about my eating in Montana. I confessed it in my first morning phone call after she got back from Maine, figuring she would either tell me I had to find another sponsor or forgive me.

I attempted to explain. "I think I needed to see myself in the food, needed to remind myself of something. I went to Montana really pissed off at leaving my life, you know? I have life on the one hand, and food on the other. And food is stronger than I am. It's like I live in a tiny room, like *No Exit*. There's me, and there's food. I can *think* it's me and life—a boy or writing or the office or being thin and wearing cool clothes—but it's really and always just me and the food. Too much of it or the right food, it doesn't matter. It will always be me and the food before any of the other stuff gets in. And it will only get in for a while. I'll have to eat again and so life has to leave for a little bit while I do that. Or I can eat everything I want and there won't be any room for the other stuff. I needed to see that. I don't know if I get it, but I got a good close look at it."

"How many recoveries do you think you have in you, Frances?" she asked. "I see you breaking your food plan in worse ways each time. This is a progressive disease and you're living it."

"I know," I sighed. "I have my life, and I have a disease. I'll eat what I'm supposed to today, I'll get to a meeting, make a phone call. What else can I do?"

"Nothing," she relented with a sigh. "You're doing the right things. You know what to do."

I told her the truth of what I'd done and reported its consequences.

I was tired. That day I did not want to fight. I wanted to wake up the next morning and be the same person I was the night before. I wanted a pearl necklace of such days, in which I was doing Frances things and reacting in Frances ways, consistently, whole and clean, so that "life's terms" came *at* me, rather than issuing from the Planet of Fat's first rule—*why try?*—or transmogrifying me into someone else's—a boy's, a boss's, a clothing designer's, my family's, food's—idea of a girl.

How many recoveries did I think I had in me? None. I'd never recovered, and I certainly didn't get thin by yanking the wherewithal out of myself. What I'd gotten came from other people: Katie, Nora, Bridget, Pam, Jennifer. My brother would call it God.

The question was, how many recoveries for me were out *there*?

I started my intergalactic quest with a million quaking pangs, of regret and of the body, earned fear that I would fail, and enough hope to try anyway. That day I thought maybe there were a thousand recoveries for me out there. The proportions of hope and hurt had been reversed.

It was five-thirty in the morning when I finished my conversation with Bridget. We both knew what I would eat that day. The food was bought and prepared, I had only to assemble and eat it. That was the one thing I could count on that day if I let it. I decided to let it. Who knew? Maybe the Catholic Boy would rub my back or I would sell a book or write a good sentence. Anything could happen.

That's the trick. Be unassailably and unflappably braced for whatever happens. It took 167 pounds, as of that morning, to get to the precipice at the foot of Mount Reynolds, but *I*, the Frances who had wanted to be right there for forty-five years and the Frances who had earned the moment, had felt the complete glory of it. Maybe size didn't matter as much as my heart and my own twisty way of looking at the world, and I knew, because the ill effects of food were still cycling sourly through my body, that my heart and mind were at their best when my eating was meted and defined. It was the only way to keep the white blaze of Jackson Glacier, blinding across the valley, a part of me.

Next year, I would be sure-footed enough to cross that valley. It would be more than enough.

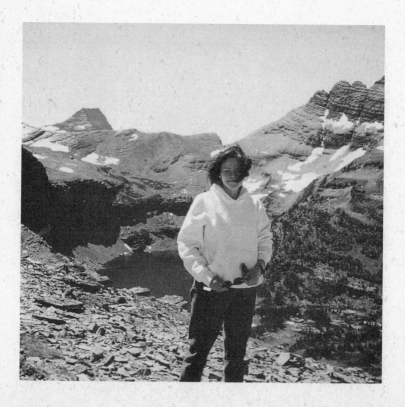

ACKNOWLEDGMENTS

This book and I have been a group project, assembled by many people. I will be haunted by guilt that someone's name has to come first, so let me start by acknowledging GlaxoSmithKline, Pfizer, and Eli Lilly & Company, and Sheila Kaplan and Lori Plutchek, who introduced us.

Showers of thanks to my first and last lines of defense, the Stepford Wives, especially Katie, Bridget, Jennifer, Nora, Pam, Christy, Tracy, Amy. You know who you are. You've shown me how to sit on my hands long enough to be myself. Thanks to all the Rooms.

Jim and Brenda Kuffel read this in email forty-two times, a number that is only exceeded by how many times Jimmie has had to dig my car out of the snow. You know who I am: I hope I'll get better.

Fredi Friedman dropped her chopsticks to say, "You have to write this story, Frances!" when I kidded about a forty-page joke book called *Passing for Thin*. Your unceasing enthusiasm, advice, and encouragement in being a writer and being an agent have kept me dog-paddling forward. I can't thank you enough for the deadlines and for taking this project—and me—in hand. Suzanne Oaks was the acquiring editor who believed in the book and my ability to do it; Becky Cole is the amazing wizardess who walked me through the process. Becky is always right. I believe in you.

Thanks to Shirley Qian, Mennary McNambe, Ella Shalmiyev, Tyrone Traylor, and Justin DeNino—the pros who polished my thinitude into a style of my own. And good God, I have friends—lots of friends! Isn't that amazing? They listened and listened and listened and read and encouraged. Jennifer Bausch, Anna Del Vecchio, Cynthia Gralla, Bob Hamilton, David Harvey, John Lucas, Tom Mitz, Lee Reilly, Tracy Sherrod, Carol Smith, and Moira Sullivan: I'm taking a year's vow of silence in order to let *you* talk.

A lump-in-my-throat thanks to Jeff Schult and Phillip DePoy. You know for what.

The Montana Gang kept me aspiring. Thanks to Fred Haefele, Peter Stark, and Jim and Lois Welch. And last—because someone has to be—thanks to Jonathan Bishop, who kept finding the novels in my letters. You didn't let me forget.

Frances Kuffel found herself in a new world when she lost half her body size. Experiences most people have had by the time they've reached adulthood—dating and heartbreak, following their ambitions with confidence, making a home and identifying their community—were daunting first-time challenges that she had to negotiate, with outside help and advice, one at a time.

If you're part of a reading group, the following questions about food and eating, body image, and authenticity may spark an even more lively discussion by highlighting key passages, exploring underlying themes and motifs, and helping you relate this memoir to your own life.

1. Did Frances's descriptions of eating and her relationship with food make you think about things you rely on that might be dangerous buffers or substitutions?

2. Has your body shaped your life? Why or why not, and how?

3. How much has popular culture affected your attitude toward your body?

4. Have you ever had a defining moment in which you realized something fundamental about the way you have lived your life? How did you act on the realization?

5. Why do you think a twelve-step program was successful for Frances when other diets and methods had failed?

6. Frances criticizes "fat serenity," the philosophy that advocates accepting one's body at a larger size, as unreasonable. Why couldn't she accept her size? Should "sizism" be a civil rights movement in the way that feminism, gay rights, and racial equality have been?

7. Why does Kuffel spend so little time on the actual diet she followed?

8. Frances enlists a number of advisors in the course of the book, relying on them to tell her what to eat, how to dress and wear her hair, guide her free time, how to think and feel about herself. Does this make her a weak person? On whom do you rely and for what?

9. What role does "passing" play in the author's account of her newly thin body? Have you ever felt you were only "passing" for/as something? Does the feeling of passing make you less authentic?

10. Kuffel admits that "*I* don't really like fat people much." Why would a formerly obese person have such a prejudice? What do you think about fat people?

11. Frances writes that "finishing is not success." Does she find success in the course of the book? Beyond finishing a project, how do you define success?

12. Which do you think is the "real" Frances Kuffel, the fat or the thin one? Do you think there are aspects of obesity she was grateful for after she lost weight? If you were to accomplish something you'd always wanted, how would it change you and what of yourself would you want to keep from "before"?

13. Frances finds an identity to inhabit from her two boyfriends' neat categorizations of why they liked her. The Boy from Connecticut found her beautiful and funny, while The Catholic Boy thought she was pretty, smart, and nice. Have your romantic involvements given you a better sense of yourself? Is there anything wrong with that?

14. Why does Frances begin to eat in the last two chapters?

15. How would you describe the "note" on which the book ends?

NOTES

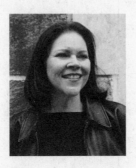

ABOUT THE AUTHOR

Frances Kuffel is a literary agent who has published poems and short stories in literary journals such as *Triquarterly*, *The Georgia Review*, *Glimmer Train*, *Prairie Schooner*, and *The Massachusetts Review*. A native of Missoula, Montana, she currently makes her home in Brooklyn, New York.